"Michael succeeds in bringing to life the day to day living with epilepsy and the personal drama of brain surgery, recovery and eventual triumph. His story told with such vibrant and honest insight, is an engaging document of struggle against adversity. It will be a source of inspiration and comfort to patients out there, and especially to those afflicted with epilepsy."

—**Dr. Itzhak Fried, professor of neurosurgery, UCLA**

"Michael's inspiring tale underscores the transformative power of perseverance and the profound impact of embracing new beginnings with courage and conviction."

—**Rob Bernshteyn, former CEO, Coupa Software**

"King has a charismatic story that aches to understand the precarious act of being alive. It's the threat of a foreshortened life that gives this book such heat. He wrote it for all of us so we never forget: today is a great day because we're all still here."

—**Joshua Mohr, author of *Model Citizen***

"Michael, your courage in facing brain surgery is truly remarkable. Thank you for bravely sharing your journey with us—it's a testament to your strength and resilience."

—**Dr. Paul Mullin, former neurologist, UCLA**

"Michael's humorous and heart-wrenching account of living with severe epilepsy is one of courage and success. From us, your medical team, thank you for your trust and for allowing us the honor of playing a part in such an important chapter of your life."

—**Dr. Sandra Dewar, epilepsy nurse specialist**

"When you learn about Michael's story, and the challenges he had to overcome, you realize what has made him so inspirational and such a good friend to many."

—Greg Ott, former CMO, Demandbase

"I've known Michael since we were in grade school together. His story is a testament to resilience, friendship, and the transformative power of grabbing life's opportunities in the face of adversity."

—Dave Yarnold, former CEO, ServiceMax

"This powerful memoir hits home for me as a father whose daughter also faces the challenges of epilepsy. Michael's journey from living with epilepsy to overcoming it through surgery is nothing short of inspiring. His story shows the resilience of the human spirit and reminds us all that there is hope, even in the toughest of battles."

—Tom Grubb, marketing executive

BE THERE WHEN I RETURN

A MEMOIR OF EPILEPSY, LOVE, AND SUCCESS

MICHAEL KING

SPARKPRESS

Published by SparkPress, a BookSparks imprint,
A division of SparkPoint Studio, LLC
Phoenix, Arizona, USA, 85007
www.gosparkpress.com

Published 2025
Printed in the United States of America

Print ISBN: 978-1-68463-298-5
E-ISBN: 978-1-68463-299-2
Library of Congress Control Number: 2024922573

Interior design and typeset by Katherine Lloyd, The DESK

"The two most important days in your life
are the day you are born
and the day you find out why."
—*Mark Twain*

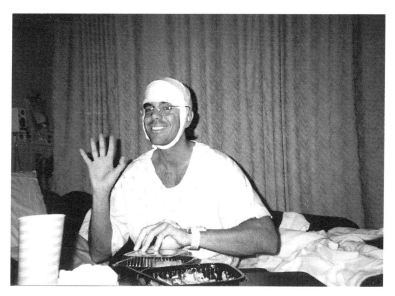

UCLA Medical Center – December 1997

ABOUT EPILEPSY

- According to the World Health Organization, epilepsy is the most common severe brain disorder worldwide, with no age, racial, social class, nationality, or geographic boundaries.
- **65 million:** Number of people around the world who have epilepsy.
- **3.4 million:** Number of people in the United States who have epilepsy.
- **45,000:** Number of children under the age of 15 who develop epilepsy each year.
- **470,000:** Number of children in the United States who have epilepsy.
- **1 in 26:** Ratio of people in the United States who will develop epilepsy at some point in their lifetime.
- **Between 4 and 10 out of 1,000:** Ratio of people on earth who live with active seizures at any one time.
- **150,000:** Number of new cases of epilepsy in the United States each year.
- **One-third:** Fraction of people with epilepsy who live with uncontrollable seizures because no available medicines work for them.
- **1 in 1,000:** Number of people who die each year from SUDEP (sudden unexpected death in epilepsy). This means that each year in the United States, there are about 3,000 deaths due to SUDEP (neurologists suspect that figure is conservative).
- **6 out of 10:** Number of people with epilepsy where the cause is unknown.
- **MST (Multiple Subpial Transection) surgery:** An alternative type of surgery used if seizures begin in a region of the brain that can't be removed safely. This would include areas in the brain that control speech or movement.
- **Funding for epilepsy:** Not enough

CHAPTER 1

FEBRUARY 1997, Los Angeles, California. Museum Terrace Apartments—6th and Curson. I walked down the hallway of my apartment carrying a folding chair, my JVC boombox, and two Corona beers. I opened the door that read ROOF ACCESS and walked up one flight of stairs to the roof.

Besides the swimming pool, the rooftop was one of my favorite places in the building. I walked over to its west side, unfolded my chair, turned on my boombox, and hit Play. Bruce Springsteen's "Human Touch" began to play as I popped one of the Coronas and sat down in my chair to enjoy the end of another sunny day in Los Angeles.

As "Human Touch" finished, "Better Days" began to play. I reached over and turned up the volume as I took the last sip of my beer. I placed the empty bottle on the ground, pushed myself up off my chair, and took a stroll around the rooftop to take in all the fantastic views of Los Angeles: to the north, the Hollywood sign; to the east, downtown Los Angeles; to the south, Baldwin Hills. Walking around the roof, I reflected on my last eleven years.

A smile came to my face as I thought about the people I had met in LA since moving there from Daly City, California—all the fun times I'd had. Box seats at Dodger Stadium as Kirk Gibson limped around the bases after hitting a walk-off home run in Game 1 of the 1988 World Series. Meeting Shaquille O'Neal during his rookie year while bartending at a nightclub in Century City (man, his hands were big). Standing in the front row at China Club in Hollywood as Elton John jumped onstage and played for forty minutes. Bartending at the Hard Rock in LA as a twenty-one-year-old Harry Connick Jr. performed with Tony Bennett at a *Spin* magazine party. Noticing that Bruce Springsteen was standing across from me as I flipped through videos at Tower Video on Sunset.

I returned to the west side of the building—which overlooked the La Brea Tar Pits and the Los Angeles County Museum of Art—and closed my eyes, feeling the sun's warmth on my face. The fun times of living in

BE THERE WHEN I RETURN

Los Angeles started to fade out of my mind, and the living hell I had been going through over the past five years began to take over. I was fighting a losing battle trying to control my epilepsy—a condition that had appeared one day out of nowhere and didn't seem inclined to go away.

Epilepsy was getting the best of me. I felt like a human guinea pig as my doctor tried to figure out the correct combination of medications to control my seizures. And those medications? They had a ton of side effects. Five years earlier, I'd been constantly on the go; I would throw my bike in my car, drive to Santa Monica, and then ride "The Strand" down to Redondo Beach and back. Now, I always felt tired. Every day, my body was drained of energy. I felt worthless. And none of the drugs that were making me feel that way were actually working to control my seizures.

My breathing accelerated as I thought about what my life might look like ten years from now if I continued to have seizures. I was a thirty-six-year-old bartender, living paycheck to paycheck, who was still trying to break into the entertainment industry after a decade of efforts. My credit card debt was growing larger every month. With my seizures, I had a challenging time keeping a steady job. When I told potential employers that I had epilepsy, I did not get hired. If I did not disclose my condition to an employer and had a seizure on the job, they thought I was on drugs or crazy and fired me.

Five years earlier, when I'd noticed someone looking at me, it had made me feel good. I would think they recognized me from my bartending job or thought I looked like an actor from a television show or movie. When someone stared at me now, it made me feel uncomfortable—I was paranoid that they thought I was on drugs or a weirdo. Many days, I felt better just staying in bed at my apartment than venturing into the world; at least there, no one would stare at me and think something was wrong with me. I knew I was not the same person I'd been before the epilepsy came along.

I inched closer to the rooftop's edge. I reached out my right foot and cautiously nudged a small rock. I followed its eight-story descent until it collided with the unforgiving cement below.

I thought about what my life might look like if I never got my driver's license back. Would I have to ask friends to pick me up and drive me around forever? Was even that an option anymore? The people I'd thought of as friends did not return my calls anymore. Would I have to take public transportation for the rest of my life?

And what about my amazing girlfriend? We'd been living together for three years. She was a beautiful, intelligent woman. She could have any guy she wanted. The two of us had been through a lot together, and she kept telling me she would never leave me, but I was sure she didn't see a bright future with a guy like me. I felt that time was running out on our relationship.

And I loved kids—wanted a family. Would I be able to have children? Would they have epilepsy? Would I be able to hold my baby without the fear of having a seizure while holding them?

When I thought about what my life might look like in ten years, the picture wasn't pretty.

I took another step closer to the edge.

My toes hung over open space as "Better Days" continued to blast from my boombox. I looked down onto Curson Avenue and wiped the tears from my face as the sky turned a flaming orangey-pink color.

My heart racing, my life began to flash in front of me.

As a kid—pretending I was San Francisco Giants pitcher Juan Marichal as I played "Strike Out" for hours at Thomas Edison Elementary School with my buddies Chris and John; working at my dad's sporting goods store, Flying Goose; closing my eyes as I sat in the back seat of my parents' car and repeating to myself, *Please let there be a red light on Columbus*, as we drove up Broadway to my aunt and uncle's house in San Francisco's North Beach neighborhood (sometimes my wish came true, and I saw the lady dancing in the cage atop one of the strip clubs next to Big Al's and Condor Club).

In high school—meatball sandwich on Thursdays at Herb's Deli on Taraval; racing my 1976 Chevy Camaro down the Great Highway and Brotherhood Way; seeing AC/DC at the Old Waldorf in San Francisco for only $3 with my buddy John; late nights at Toto's Pizza with my buddy Jay (I put on twenty pounds over that summer; the pot didn't help).

In junior college—meeting my lifelong friend Bob while attending Cañada Junior College; playing baseball at Cañada JC with two future Major League players, Harold Reynolds and Bob Melvin; sneaking second-year 49ers quarterback Joe Montana into the over-capacity Balboa Café through one of the sliding windows.

At St. Mary's College—Bob and I engraving our names on a plaque in a park in Moraga, California; hearing a voice call out, "MK!" on graduation day as I made my way across the stage to receive my diploma, and turning to see my childhood friend Chris holding a bottle of champagne meant for me.

After college—going to the 1984 MLB All-Star Game at Candlestick Park with my dad; carrying Bob piggyback at 2:00 a.m., singing "New York, New York" as we walked down the middle of Greenwich Street in San Francisco after a night partying at "The Triangle."

As the sun set into the ocean, the sky underwent a breathtaking transformation, splashing vibrant colors across the horizon. The joys of my life suddenly faded, and the darkness of the last five years' struggles overtook my inner thoughts again.

I lowered my head. My body quivered uncontrollably. Tears rolled down my face and dropped to the gravel beneath me. I gazed down at my toes, dangling precariously over the edge of the building. I shut my eyes and whispered a silent plea—

I just want to feel better.

CHAPTER 2

F IVE YEARS EARLIER: Monday, April 6, 1992. Marabella Apartments on 6th and Detroit in Los Angeles—the fifth place I'd lived in since my buddy Chris helped me load all my stuff into a U-Haul truck and I moved to LA in January of 1986.

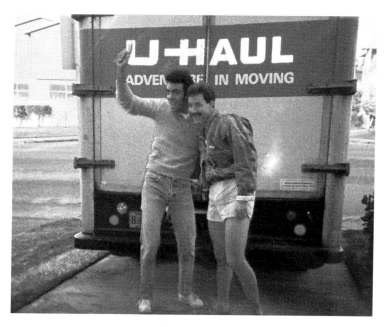

Ready to move to LA

This apartment was my favorite of the five because it was across the street from the King King—*the* place to listen to great rhythm and blues music by local musicians. The house band, The Red Devils, played on Monday nights, and well-known musicians and celebrities often jumped onstage to jam with the band. I'd seen Bruce Willis play harmonica on that stage, and Mick Jagger had shown up one night and performed the Bo Diddley classics "Who Do You Love?" and "Blues with a Feeling" with the Devils.

Since it was early April, that meant only one thing to a sports fan like me: March Madness and the NCAA Men's Basketball Tournament. After watching Duke upset Kentucky in the East Regional Final in a game many would, even decades later, consider the greatest college basketball game of all time, my roommate Tim and I had invited two buddies, Rich and Alex, to come over and watch the championship game between Duke and Michigan.

We'd ordered a large pizza and had a fridge full of Coronas, so we were all set.

Tim and I had met a few years earlier when he became a manager at the Hard Rock in LA, where I worked. We would head up to Roxbury on Sunset many nights after work, and since I'd successfully leveraged "club courtesy" while working at the Hard Rock in San Francisco to get into the clubs in San Francisco—The Oasis, Club D8, Trocadero Transfer—I decided to try it in LA. It worked like a charm; Tim and I never had to wait outside with the large crowd trying to get picked to get into Roxbury or any other hot clubs in LA—Glam Slam (Prince's nightclub), BarOne, The Gate, Vertigo. All I had to do was make eye contact with one of the doormen—which was easy, since I was six feet, four inches tall.

I had always believed the saying *It's not what you know, it's who you know*, but I started to change my philosophy on that saying during this time; I started to think that maybe the most important thing wasn't who you knew but rather who knew you. Later in my life, I would only become further convinced on this point.

The first half of the championship game ended with Michigan ahead 31–30. About halfway through the second half, Duke called a time-out. The network went to a commercial break, and a commercial for the upcoming Masters golf tournament started to play.

"Hey!" Alex called out to me.

The tone of his voice startled me. I looked over at him and was momentarily unsure where I was, or who the other two guys in the room were. I felt like I was in a fog.

"Hey," Alex repeated. "You okay?"

It took me a few seconds to respond, but finally my senses returned to me. "What?" I said. "Yeah, I'm fine. Why?"

Rich chuckled, his expression a peculiar mix of amusement and bewilderment, as he asked, "Why did you do that?"

"Do what?" His words utterly baffled me, and all the questioning was starting to wear on my patience.

"Man, I know you like golf, but you don't need to get that excited about a fucking tournament," Alex said, enjoying a good laugh with Rich.

I looked over at Tim, still trying to get my bearings.

Tim stared at me, trying to figure out if I was serious or playing around. He finally smiled, sipped his beer, and playfully asked, "What the fuck was that all about? Are you fucking with us?"

I had reached the end of my rope with their questions. "What?" I snapped. "What the fuck are you guys talking about?"

I looked over at the TV, and the game was back on. The last thing I remembered was the beginning of the commercial for the Masters golf tournament. I reached down and picked up my Corona, took a big sip, and concentrated on the game. And I never thought a second time about what had just happened—not until much later, anyway.

CHAPTER 3

SIX MONTHS EARLIER, I'd started dating someone new. I'd met her where I met most of the girls I dated: the Hard Rock Café.

It was the summer of 1991, and it was a typical Saturday night at the Hard Rock; the bar was four deep, and there was a line around the corner to get in. The bartenders, me included, were moving frantically to keep up with the nonstop drink orders. I'd become used to lining up kamikazes and Coronas for actors like Rob Lowe, Emilio Estevez, and Charlie Sheen by that point. That night, I was posted at the service station on the circular bar's backside. The drink orders from the servers felt like they would never end.

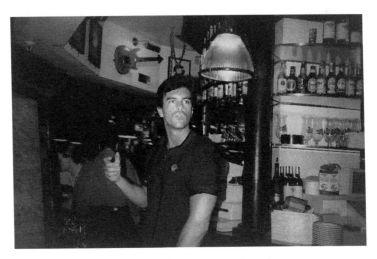

Behind the bar – LA Hard Rock

Finally, there was a bit of a break, and I was able to come up for air.

Steve, a busser I was friendly with, approached the service station with a big grin on his face. "Did you see the girl at table twenty-five?"

I looked up at the table and noticed two people sitting there: a guy and a woman. The guy was well dressed and looked like he was in his late thirties. The woman looked like she was in her late twenties. She had a beautiful face and long brunette hair. The guy's body language made it hard to tell if they were a couple or just friends. He had positioned his back against the wall and stretched his legs along the bench. He was sipping his drink and taking in all the action at the sunken bar below, as if he was unaware that a beautiful woman was seated right across from him.

As I looked at her, she slowly turned and caught me staring. I smiled at her, and she cracked a small smile. Since the guy was not paying attention to her, he never noticed her looking at me. I quickly grabbed a napkin and a pen and wrote, *Is he your boyfriend/husband . . . Yes or No? If no, would you like to have a drink sometime? – Michael.* I handed the napkin and pen to Steve and said, "When he goes to the bathroom, give this to her."

I went back to making drinks, occasionally glancing at her table, hoping the guy would go to the bathroom. Finally, I saw him getting up; as soon as he was gone, I looked at Steve and motioned for him to go over to her.

I watched as he handed her the napkin and pen and pointed down to me. She looked down, read the napkin, and then quickly wrote on it and handed it back to Steve.

The anticipation was killing me as he returned to the bar. He handed me the napkin, and I quickly unfolded it—and the word *HUSBAND* jumped off the napkin.

Deflated, I crumpled up the napkin and threw it in the garbage.

Later that night, they exited the table and walked down the steps to the restaurant's lower level. I could not keep my eyes off her as she descended the steps. She was beautiful. She wore a hot-pink miniskirt, matching top, and white high-heel pumps. As she got closer, I noticed her toned, bronzed body. Her top was short and showed off her fit stomach.

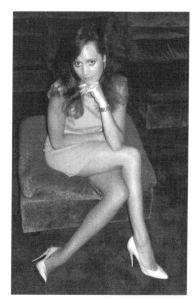

Donnita – Pink dress

She walked three steps behind her husband as they walked up the ramp toward the exit. There was zero affection. No holding hands. Nothing. She turned and smiled at me just before the door closed behind her.

CHAPTER 4

THREE MONTHS LATER, I was behind the bar again, making a large order of drinks, when the barback approached me and said, "There's a girl on the other side of the bar asking for you. She said her name is Bonnita."

"Bonnita? I don't know anyone named Bonnita." I brushed him off and went back to concentrating on filling the order.

"Okay, but she's fucking hot!" he said as he walked away.

Well, that got my attention.

I quickly finished making the drinks and headed around the bar to see this mystery woman. I stopped dead in my tracks when I realized it was the napkin woman.

She was standing behind two women seated at the bar; by the looks of it, they knew each other. As I got closer, I could see her from head to toe. She was just as beautiful as I remembered.

"Well, hello there," I said.

She smiled. "Hello."

She introduced me to the two women seated at the bar—her sister-in-law, Terri, and Terri's daughter, who was visiting from Ohio.

She then moved closer to the bar and introduced herself. "Hi. My name is Donnita."

"Nice to meet you." I shook her hand gently—more of a caress than a shake.

I dropped off three drinks in front of them, then went back to doing my job—walking around the bar, talking to customers, and filling drink orders.

About thirty minutes later, I noticed three empty glasses in front of Donnita, who was now seated at the bar with her friends. I walked over to them and asked if they wanted another round.

"We're ready to close our bill, actually," Donnita said.

"No need," I said. "The drinks are on me." As bartenders, we could comp a certain number of drinks every night.

"Where you guys going?" I asked as they stood up off the barstools.

"Chippendales!" Terri's daughter cried out gleefully.

Terri and Donnita just smiled; clearly, she was looking forward to that part of her trip.

Donnita leaned over to me. "Did you ever bartend at Chippendales? You look so familiar."

Her question threw me off guard for a second. I looked at her and finally answered, "Yes, I did. I worked there back in '86 and '87."

When I'd first started working at the Hard Rock, they'd only given me two day shifts a week, so I'd taken a second job bartending at Chippendales. During my first shift at Chippendales, I'd learned two things: (1) Waxing your chest hurts like hell; (2) You shouldn't be surprised to see a woman walk into the men's bathroom with one or two Chippendales employees.

Donnita quickly turned to Terri. "I told you he worked at Chippendales!"

Terri's daughter was getting antsy. "Come on," she urged, "let's go!"

They finally said their goodbyes and made their way to the exit. I could not keep my eyes off Donnita as she made her way up the ramp. Just before leaving, she turned and waved. I smiled at her and patted my heart with my right hand. I hoped I'd see her again soon.

I enjoyed being single and working at one of the hottest bars in LA. I never wanted to be one of those guys who had a girlfriend but messed around on the side. I'd learned that lesson early on, while working as a barback at the Balboa Café in San Francisco after graduating from college. During the early '80s, it was one of three bars/restaurants at the intersection of Greenwich and Fillmore (the other two were Dartmouth Social Club and Pierce Street Annex), and on weekends hundreds of people descended on that intersection. Some people called it "The Bermuda Triangle"—or just "The Triangle" for short—because it was a place where singles suddenly disappeared into the night. While I was there, one of the bartenders at the Balboa was dating one of the waitresses. At work one night, they started arguing, loudly—the waitress had just found out he was cheating on her. Their tenure at the Balboa ended when she threw a tray of drinks at him that busy Saturday night.

I didn't want to be that guy. I wasn't ready to settle down either. And

I'd always told myself that I would never get involved with a married woman. But I could not stop thinking about Donnita—and I soon learned that she felt the same way.

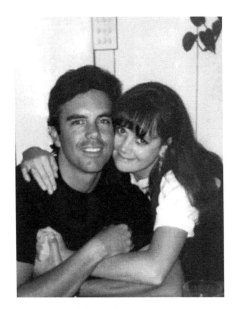

Me and Donnita

OVER THE NEXT SIX MONTHS, I learned a lot about Donnita. She'd grown up in Sylmar, California. She had three sisters: Lisa, Sharon, and Becky. When she was eighteen, her parents and her youngest sister, Becky, had moved to Wenatchee, Washington, for her dad's new job. She'd decided to stay in LA at the family house in Sylmar and paid the mortgage with the help of roommates. She'd won the Miss Hollywood Hemisphere beauty pageant. She'd toured the world playing softball for The Hollywood Cover Girls softball team.

And she'd gotten married in 1989.

We laughed one day as we reminisced about my clever move, having Steve deliver my note to her that first night. She said she was nervous when her husband returned to the table, thinking he might have seen her talking to the busser, but he said nothing. He just sat back down, leaned back on the wooden bench, put his feet up, and started surveying the bar crowd.

"As he sipped his drink, he looked at me, smiled, and said, 'I'm the best-looking guy here!' I snickered under my breath—he's always saying things like that to me—and he glared at me and said, 'I'm more beautiful as a man than you will ever be as a woman.'"

My eyes widened; I couldn't believe he would say something like that to her.

"As he took another sip of his drink, I shook my head in disgust and said, 'You want to see my idea of a beautiful man?' He gave me this arrogant look and said, 'Sure. Go ahead. Who?' So I pointed behind the bar at you and said, 'The tall bartender with dark hair. Now that is a beautiful man!'"

I couldn't help but smile at this. It was nice to know she'd been admiring me too.

She said that her husband quickly sat up to get a better look at this so-called beautiful man. After looking at me behind the bar, he chuckled and said, "Yeah, like he would give *you* the time of day!" Then he leaned back on the wooden bench, put his feet back up, and sipped his drink.

Donnita just sat there, looked at her husband, sipped her wine, and kept her little secret to herself.

DURING THIS TIME, I also learned about the mental and physical abuse Donnita had endured from her husband. She shared with me that he would slap her in the face or punch her if she said something he did not like. He would also talk down to her, making her feel worthless and stupid.

One day, I noticed a small scar on her left temple next to her eyebrow and asked, "How did you get that?"

She reached up and touched it with her left hand. After a brief pause, she said, "He gave it to me."

Another time, when she was over at my place, she went to get up off the futon and suddenly grabbed her lower back.

"Are you okay?" I asked, concerned.

"Yeah," she said, "I'm okay."

But as she moved slowly toward my bedroom and eventually the bathroom, I could see by how she was walking that something was not right. So when she finally returned to the living room, I asked, "Did you hurt your back?"

She paused for a moment. I could tell this was a touchy subject.

It took a minute, but she finally confided in me. Her husband had come home drunk one night and kicked her in between the legs. He was wearing cowboy boots, and the tip of his boot had hit the back of her hip. Ever since, her sacroiliac had been flaring up here and there.

I was brought up with the belief that a man should never harm a woman, so I could not understand how a guy would do this to a woman he supposedly loved.

Seeing the pain she was in because of him, I felt helpless. I wished I could protect her from him.

BE THERE WHEN I RETURN

As I got to know Donnita better, she shared with me that she'd known on her wedding day, while walking down the aisle clutching her father's arm, that she was making a huge mistake. She confided in me that she kept beating herself up because she hadn't listened to her inner voice when it counted. She also shared with me that, in her mind, she had divorced her husband years ago; she was just too afraid to leave him.

Finally, in March of 1992, she drummed up the courage to leave. One day, she told her husband that she wanted to drive up the coast, get a hotel room, pray, and think things over. "I'll be back tomorrow night," she told him.

After hearing that, he walked over and picked up her purse off the table. He pulled out her wallet, took out all her credit cards, and put just one back into her wallet; then he took almost all her cash, leaving her only $40 in her wallet.

Donnita picked up her purse and the overnight bag and walked toward the front door without saying a word.

He looked at her and said, "Take as long as you need."

She was surprised that he was being nice, but she realized he knew he was losing her. He thought his paltry effort to be caring might encourage her to come home the next night and not leave him for good.

But Donnita had no plans to return home. As she got down to PCH (Pacific Coast Highway) that afternoon, she made a left and went south instead of making a right and heading north. She was never planning on going "up the coast" for the night; she was headed to Newport Beach, where her best friend lived. Earlier that day, while her husband was at the gym, she'd filled up her big suitcase with some of her belongings and put it in the trunk of her Corvette.

Donnita stayed with her best friend until April, when she moved into an apartment in Newport Beach with a roommate. On August 13, 1998, Donnita was legally divorced from her husband.

CHAPTER 5

THREE DAYS AFTER the Duke–Michigan game, I parked my car in front of Donnita's apartment in Newport Beach, grabbed my bag from my car, and made my way to her apartment. She and I planned to have dinner that evening and then go on a bike ride the following day.

After dinner, we decided to walk down to the Newport Beach Pier. Halfway along the pier, we stopped to lean against the rail and watch the sunset. I held Donnita close to me and kissed her on the cheek.

After a few minutes, we continued walking down the pier. As we watched the surfers trying to get in the last wave of the day, Donnita suddenly asked, "Why did you do that?"

I looked at her, perplexed. For a moment, I was not sure where I was. "What?" I finally answered her. "Do what?"

Donnita just looked at me, shrugged, and softly said, "Okay."

I took her by the hand, and we continued to walk down the pier.

I AWOKE EARLY the following morning. Donnita was still sleeping, so I was quiet as I got out of bed and walked to the bathroom next to her bedroom.

Suddenly, I heard her call out, "Michael!"

I looked at her blankly. I wasn't entirely sure where I was; things were a bit foggy. The last thing I remembered was washing my hands at the sink.

"Michael!" she called out again and motioned for me to get back into bed.

I looked around, orienting myself. I was standing in front of Donnita's roommate's bedroom. The bedroom door was slightly ajar, and I was standing completely naked.

"Michael! Get in here!" Again, Donnita beckoned to me.

I walked back to her bedroom and got into bed. I was lucky that her roommate was out of town.

CHAPTER 6

ON THE AFTERNOON OF APRIL 29, Tim and I ran up to the rooftop of our apartment and looked south with disbelieving eyes. Black smoke filled the sky, and we could see flames coming from burning buildings. This was the aftereffect of a jury acquitting four Los Angeles police officers for the brutal beating of Rodney King. The city looked like a war zone.

Two days later, the phone rang. It was my mom.

"Are you okay?" she asked. "I'm watching the news. One reporter said that the riots have moved north toward Wilshire and up La Brea."

"It has been crazy here, but we are fine," I reassured her. Sprawled out on the futon in my living room, I gave my mom the details of the fires and looting in the area. I told her how Tim and I had been on the roof, watching the fires, when a truck pulled up in front of Radio Shack directly across from us on La Brea. Three guys jumped out, smashed the windows, and looted the store. Tim and I just stood there, watching these guys walk out with new computers. There was looting throughout LA, so the police could not be everywhere, and everyone knew it. "Tim and I thought briefly about running across the street and grabbing a computer," I admitted, "but we decided it was a bad idea."

"Way to exercise good judgment," she said.

And then . . .

"Michael! Michael!"

I looked around, trying to figure out where that insistent voice was coming from. Everything was a bit foggy. I finally realized that I was in my bedroom, lying on my bed, and noticed the phone next to me.

"Michael!" It was my mom's voice.

I picked up the phone. "Yes?" I said casually, trying to act as if nothing had happened.

"Are you okay?" she asked.

"Yeah—yeah, I am fine." I was unsure how I'd ended up on my bed, but I continued the conversation with my mom as if nothing had happened. After this incident, I began trying to put the pieces together on what was happening, but I still never felt like anything was wrong with me.

CHAPTER 7

A WEEK AFTER things had calmed down with the LA riots, Donnita came over to my apartment to spend the weekend. She and I were watching television on the futon when the front door opened and Tim walked in, two bags of groceries in his hands.

Donnita jumped up off the futon. "Let me help you," she said, and followed him into the kitchen.

As the two of them put away groceries, they started talking. I couldn't hear what they were saying over the noise of the TV, but I could see their faces, and I could tell it wasn't the casual conversation I was used to seeing between them; it looked like they were having a serious talk. I didn't think much of it and went back to watching television.

After they put away the groceries, the two of them walked into the living room together. Tim sat in the papasan chair across from me and Donnita sat beside me on the futon, serious looks on their faces.

I looked over at Tim and then back at Donnita, chuckled, and said, "What's up?"

Donnita took a deep breath and looked at me; her eyes started to fill with tears. She then glanced at Tim. "Tim, have you ever seen Michael clap his hands like this"—she started to clap her hands together in front of her—"and then start yelling, 'Woo-hoo, woo-hoo!'" She shook her body from side to side and continued to clap her hands as she did this.

I looked over at Tim. He looked at Donnita; he could not look me in the eyes. "Yes," he said. "He did that when we watched the basketball game with Alex and Rich."

"What? What the hell are you talking about?" I shook my head. "You're telling me that when we were watching the basketball game, out of nowhere I just started clapping my hands and yelling 'Woo-hoo'? Come on!" I giggled under my breath.

"Yeah, you did!" Tim insisted. "Remember I asked you what the fuck that was all about and if you were fucking with us?"

I had heard enough; I felt overwhelmed. I got up from the futon.

Donnita jumped in, "You did that exact thing when we were at the Newport Pier too. Remember I asked you why you did that?"

"This is crazy!" I paced the floor.

Donnita motioned for me to sit down. "Come here," she said calmly. "Sit down."

I was not ready to sit down just yet.

She got up and moved over to me. "You need to go see a doctor," she said firmly. "This is not like you. Something is not right. You don't know that you are doing these things."

I turned away from her, started pacing again. "There is nothing wrong with me. I am not going to see a doctor."

She followed me. "Remember when you were at my apartment and standing naked in front of my roommate's door?"

"Yeah, so?"

She cornered me and looked me in the eye. "When you were standing there, you started yelling, "Be funky!" and thrusting your hips toward her room. You're lucky she wasn't home!"

I was having a hard time hearing this. I edged around her and continued to pace the living room floor.

"Michael, please make an appointment to see your doctor," she pleaded.

"I just had a checkup two months ago," I snapped. "I'm fine."

"Please, buddy," Tim chimed in. "Just see your doctor. I'm sure it's nothing."

"Okay . . . okay." I gave up resisting. "I'll make an appointment to go see my doctor."

"Thank you." Donnita gave me a big hug.

I still wasn't convinced what they told me was happening to me was true. I was a healthy thirty-one-year-old guy. I didn't do drugs or have a drinking problem. Whatever this was, I was sure it would eventually go away.

OVER THE NEXT month, Donnita would witness me clapping my hands and making strange noises again. Each time it happened, she would ask me if I had made an appointment to see my doctor; each time, I would devise different excuses for why I hadn't had a chance to do it yet. Once I even told Donnita I had an appointment scheduled, but the doctor had called and needed to reschedule it to a later date—a blatant lie, but I wanted her to stop hassling me about it.

Little did I know that my out-of-character actions were symptoms of a mystery that went far beyond what I or anyone else could have anticipated.

CHAPTER 8

Two months later, I arrived bright and early for my first day of training as a bartender at a new restaurant/bar in Costa Mesa, California. The grand opening loomed—it was just a month out—and everyone was bustling at lightning speed. Having been one of the original bartenders at the Hard Rock in San Francisco when it opened its doors in 1984, I was no stranger to the exhilaration of launching a new restaurant.

The banquet rooms in a nearby hotel were converted into training rooms for the different departments: bartenders and barbacks were in one room; servers, bussers, and hosts were in another; and kitchen staff were in a third.

The first week of training went smoothly. The manager reviewed the drink and food menus and then discussed what he expected from us behind the bar. During the second week of training, the manager told us there would be a group meeting with all the staff, the managers, and the general manager the following morning. The general manager would review the timeline for the restaurant's opening and other company info.

As I left our training room, I ran into Diane, a friend I'd first met when she was a waitress at the Hard Rock in LA. She was one of the many female friends I'd made while working at the Hard Rock—something my male coworkers, who didn't seem capable of having female friends without being sexually attracted to them, were always amazed by. Since Diane also lived in LA, we'd been discussing the possibility of finding an apartment in Newport Beach together now that we were going to be working in Costa Mesa. From my current place the commute would be over one hour—plus, I wanted to be closer to Donnita.

"Any luck finding a place in Newport?" I asked her.

"Yeah," she said, "I have a few places I think we should look at. Do you want to check them out after tomorrow's meeting?"

"Sure," I said, "that would be great. I'll see you tomorrow morning!"

I left for the day feeling good about my new job and new housing prospects. Everything seemed to be shaping up perfectly.

I arrived the next morning for the staff meeting feeling excited to get back behind the bar at a busy restaurant/bar. I hadn't been working for a few months—not since being let go from the Hard Rock Café in LA earlier in the year.

The room buzzed with a diverse assembly of staff members, including bar staff, servers, bussers, kitchen staff, hosts, office staff, managers, and the general manager. Diane was sitting directly across from me with the other servers. I smiled and waved to her, and she waved back.

The managers got up individually, introduced themselves, and told us about their backgrounds. After that, the general manager introduced himself and told us about his background. He then turned it over to the head of human resources, who discussed the benefits package we'd be offered. After that, they wrapped it up—the general manager got up again and instructed everyone to return to their training rooms.

Everyone except the bar manager was there when I returned to the bartender/barback room. It seemed like thirty minutes passed before he finally returned. When he did, he made a beeline to me and said, "I need to speak with you outside."

I followed him out of the room and into the hallway. "What's up?" I asked.

"Jeff wants to speak with you." Jeff was the general manager.

"Is something wrong?" I asked.

"Jeff will explain everything." The shortness of his answer worried me. What the hell was going on?

As I followed the bar manager down the hallway, I started to play out different scenarios, trying to figure out what Jeff could possibly want to speak to me about. Nothing made sense, so I finally gave up speculating and followed the bar manager into a room.

Jeff was seated in a chair when I entered the room. The bar manager motioned me to a chair across from him, and then he sat down beside him. Unclear whether this was going to be good news or bad news, I fidgeted in my chair, trying to find a comfortable spot.

Jeff looked at the bar manager, then back at me. "We hired a lot of good bartenders," he said slowly. "After taking a long, hard look at the bartenders we have hired, we feel that we do not need this many bartenders right now, and unfortunately, we have to let you go."

I just sat there for a moment and took it all in. Then I met the bar manager's gaze. "This doesn't make sense. You told me I was going to be your number one bartender."

He could not look me in the eyes.

I looked at Jeff. "What the hell is going on?"

Jeff stood up. "I'm really sorry, Michael. This was our fault. We just over-hired."

I stared at him. "Is it because of what happened at the Hard Rock? I told you guys the truth about what happened."

"No, that's not it," he said. "I'm really sorry."

I just sat there for another minute, stunned. Then, without saying another word, I got up and left the room, thinking, *What the hell just happened?*

I walked down the hall in a daze. As I passed one of the small banquet rooms, I spotted Diane inside and waved her over.

As she got closer, she saw the look on my face. "What's wrong?"

I shook my head in disbelief. "I just got fired."

She paused a moment, then asked, "Are you okay?"

"No!" I said. "I'm *not* okay. I just got fired!"

She softly touched my arm. "Michael . . . are you *okay*?"

I was baffled. "What? What are you talking about?"

She got a pained look in her eyes. "In the middle of the meeting, when the general manager was talking, you stood up and started clapping your hands loudly and then yelled, 'Woo-hoo, woo-hoo!'"

I just stood there as it hit me. *Holy shit! That is exactly what Donnita and Tim said I have been doing.* I hadn't believed them before, but it was hard not to believe them now.

Without saying a word, I spun around and started to walk away. Halfway down the hall, my walk turned into a run.

"Michael!" Diane yelled as I ran out the door.

I jumped into my car and drove off.

I went straight to Donnita's. When I got there, I jumped out of my car, sprinted into the small apartment complex, and climbed the stairs two at a time.

I was breathless and perspiring by the time I made it to her apartment. I pounded on the door and called her name. Each passing second felt like an eternity as I stood there, anxiously waiting for her to answer.

The door finally swung open. Donnita stood there, and one look at me told her that something was not right. "What's wrong?" she asked.

Overcome with emotion, I couldn't answer. I just walked past her, down the hallway, and into her room. She followed me into her bedroom and closed the door behind her. I sat on her bed and covered my face with my hands.

She sat beside me and put her arms around me. "You are scaring me. What's going on?"

I started to cry uncontrollably, my whole body shaking. She held me until the worst of it passed; only then was I finally able to look into her eyes and speak.

"I just got fired!" I howled. "You and Tim were right; there is something wrong with me. There is something wrong with me! I will make an appointment to see a doctor—I promise. I promise."

"What happened?" she asked gently.

"I did what you and Tim said I have been doing in front of everyone at our staff meeting. Everyone must think I'm on drugs or something."

"Everything is going to be okay," Donnita said, holding me tight. "Everything is going to be okay."

But it was hard to believe that was true.

CHAPTER 9

TWO WEEKS LATER, I had an appointment to see my primary care doctor at the Cedars-Sinai Medical Office. I asked Donnita to come with me. After she and I had described to my doctor what I had been doing and that I had no recollection of any of it, she immediately referred me to a neurologist.

A few weeks later, Donnita and I drove to the Cedars-Sinai Medical Office to meet with Dr. Clarke Espy. My life had started spiraling out of control, and I couldn't ignore it any longer. The episodes of forgetfulness, the sudden outbursts of emotions, and the moments of losing touch with reality had by this point become frequent companions in my day-to-day existence.

Donnita had been a pillar of support throughout this ordeal. She held my hand as we sat in the waiting room of the neurologist's office. Her fingers were trembling ever so slightly, reflecting the anxiety coursing through both of us. I could sense her worry, even if she tried to hide it with a reassuring smile. Knowing that I was not alone in this made all the difference.

Finally, the nurse called my name, breaking the tense silence in the waiting room. The nurse escorted us into an office, and we settled into the chairs facing a desk.

"Dr. Espy will be right with you," she said as she closed the door behind her.

A few minutes later, there was a knock on the door, and Dr. Espy entered the room. We shook hands and exchanged pleasantries. His eyes radiated empathy as he began to ask me about my medical history, my parents' medical history, and whether I'd ever sustained any concussions or head injuries that might be connected to the peculiar occurrences my primary care doctor had shared with him.

He then turned his attention to Donnita. "Can you describe to me what you have witnessed Michael doing?"

Donnita went into detail about each incident—the one on the Newport Beach Pier, the one in her apartment when her roommate was out of town, and more. For me, her every word hung heavy in the air, each a struggle to grasp and comprehend.

"Do you remember any of this, Michael?" Dr. Espy asked when Donnita was done.

"No," I said. "I don't."

Donnita seemed to sense my distress; she reached over and held my hand.

Dr. Espy looked down at his pad of paper and then at me. "The first time you did anything like this was when you were watching a basketball game with your roommate and two friends?"

"Yes." My whole body was tense as I answered him. Donnita rubbed my arm.

Dr. Espy had heard enough; he decided to put me through a complete neurological examination.

The first step was to test my mental acuity. He asked if I knew where I was, my name, my birth date, and what day it was.

Next was my motor function. He had me push and pull against his hands with my legs and arms. He then checked my balance by having me close my eyes and gently pushing me from side to side.

Next up was the cranial nerve test. I had to close my eyes and identify a smell, and then I had to follow a light in his hand from side to side. He then had me turn my head from side to side against his resistance.

A coordination test was next. I had to walk on a line on the floor, close my eyes, and touch my nose and then my eyes.

After that, we did a sensory test. Dr. Espy touched my arms and legs with an alcohol swab and asked whether I felt it.

Last was my plantar reflex test, which involved the doctor stimulating the soles of my feet with a blunt instrument to judge my reflexes. My toes went down, which was good.

I passed every test, so the doctor recommended a brain CT (computed tomography) scan—which, he explained, used a combination of X-rays and a computer to create pictures of your organs, bones, and other tissues and showed more detail than a regular X-ray.

As Dr. Espy was writing down notes about my CT scan, I blurted out, "Do I have Tourette's or something like that?"

"No," he said decisively.

"So then what's wrong with me?"

"The CT scan should give us more information," he said, and refused to say any more.

A few weeks later, the results of my CT scan came back normal, so Dr. Espy scheduled me for an awake and sleep electroencephalogram (EEG), a test used to evaluate the electrical activity in the brain. Brain cells communicate with each other through electrical impulses called brain waves; an EEG can help doctors assess whether there are abnormal patterns in those impulses.

A week later, Dr. Espy's office called to set up an appointment for me to discuss the EEG findings. Donnita came with me again.

"Your EEG showed a spike and slowing in the right parietal lobe of your brain," he told me as soon as we were settled in his office.

"Parietal lobe?" I repeated, unfamiliar with the term.

"The parietal lobes are located near the back and top of the head," he explained. "The parietal lobe is vital for sensory perception and integration, including taste, hearing, sight, touch, and smell."

"So what does that mean?" I asked.

"I believe you have complex partial epilepsy," he said somberly. "Complex partial epilepsy refers to seizures that impair awareness and usually start in one part of the brain, most often in the temporal lobe or frontal lobe. They can also start in other areas too. Complex partial epilepsy starting in the temporal lobes is the most common type of epilepsy for adults."

"Epilepsy?" I said incredulously. "I can't have epilepsy. I don't fall on the ground and shake uncontrollably."

I had heard of epilepsy, but all I knew about it was what I'd seen in the movies or on television. I couldn't have epilepsy. Never in a million years had I imagined it would become my reality. I looked over at Donnita and found her eyes filled with a mixture of fear, concern, and unwavering support—as well as the same shock I was feeling.

"I know this is a lot to take in, Michael, but I believe we have identified the cause of your behavior," Dr. Espy said. "Medication should be able to control your seizures."

I left that day with a prescription for Tegretol, an anti-seizure drug that at the time was used as a first-line medication for generalized and partial complex seizure disorders. Some common side effects of Tegretol are nausea, dizziness, drowsiness, dry mouth, loss of balance, and vomiting. Dr. Espy instructed me to take 100 milligrams at night for three days, then gradually increase the dose over the next two weeks until I got up to 200 milligrams per night.

I couldn't believe that I, a man in his prime, had just been handed this diagnosis. It felt as if life was playing a cruel joke on me. I had so many plans and dreams; now they all seemed fragile and out of reach.

Oh, and Dr. Espy also wanted to conduct one last test—an MRI.

CHAPTER 10

An MRI scan uses a large magnet, radio waves, and a computer to create a detailed cross-sectional image of internal organs and structures. The MRI I was about to undergo would produce images of blood flow to specific brain areas.

The scanner before me resembled a large tube with a table in the middle, allowing the patient—me—to slide in.

Before sending me in, the technician reminded me that I had to remain perfectly still once I was inside the tube. "Any movement will disrupt the images, much like a camera trying to photograph a moving object," he warned me.

I lay as still as I could as the scanner emitted its loud banging noises, telling myself all the while, *Don't move . . . don't move.*

The following week, Dr. Espy had me return to his office to discuss my MRI results.

"It's all good news here," he informed Donnita and me. "There were no abnormal areas of enhancement, and your ventricles are normal in size and shape and show no evidence of compression or displacement of the midline structures. There's no extra-axial fluid collection, and no areas of abnormal signal intensity within your brain."

"So . . . I don't have epilepsy?" I asked hopefully.

He shook his head. "Given the spiking and slowing in your right parietal lobe, I still feel you have some form of epilepsy, unfortunately. Have you been taking the Tegretol?"

"Yes, I have."

"Have you had any incidents since your last appointment?"

I glanced over at Donnita, reluctant to answer. "Yes," I said. "I had one two days ago."

Dr. Espy looked at Donnita. "What happened?"

"We went to El Capitan Theatre to see a movie," she said. "We were seated in the front row of the balcony section. About ten minutes into the movie, Michael stood up, clapped his hands, and yelled, 'Woo-hoo!'—and then turned to me, reached down, lifted me from my chair, and started twirling me around dangerously close to the edge of the balcony. Then he placed me back in my chair, sat down, and acted as if nothing had happened. It was like he had superhuman strength."

"Do you remember that happening, Michael?" Dr. Espy asked.

Staring down at my lap, I softly said, "No."

Dr. Espy jotted down some notes. "Okay," he said. "I want you to continue taking the Tegretol, and I want you to return in a few weeks so we can do a liver panel and check the medication's levels in your blood."

He stood up then, but I was not ready to leave yet. I had to ask him the question that had been puzzling both Donnita and me for weeks.

"How do I suddenly start having seizures out of the blue one day?" I asked. "I am thirty-two years old and healthy. Where did it come from?"

Dr. Espy sat back down in his chair. "Well, you were most likely born with it, and it has been dormant all this time. For some reason, it's decided to surface now."

"You should tell Dr. Espy about what happened at the Hard Rock," Donnita said. "I think it could have something to do with what is happening with you."

Dr. Espy leaned forward in his seat. "What happened at the Hard Rock?"

I took a deep breath and began. I told him I had worked for the Hard Rock for eight years and had been behind the LA Hard Rock bar since 1986, when I moved to LA. One night, I made a mistake and did not ring up a drink at the end of my shift, and I was fired the next night when I showed up for work. This was the first time that anything like that had happened to me. No write-up, no warning, nothing—just *You're fired.* I told him how emotional I was as I told my fellow bartenders, bussers, and servers that I'd just been fired. After many hugs and tears, I finally approached the ramp leading to the main entrance. My breathing accelerated as I walked up to the front door. I loved working there. I stopped and tried to catch my breath as I reached for one of the large golden doors. The next thing I knew, I was sitting on my bed. I had no idea how I'd gotten home. If someone had asked me if I'd taken Beverly to La Brea or San Vicente to 6th Street to get home, I could not have told them.

After taking all this in, Dr. Espy asked, "When did this happen?"

"Two weeks before I was watching the basketball game with my buddies and had that first episode I told you about."

Dr. Espy nodded thoughtfully. "It's possible that experience could have had some effect on you."

This exchange made it clear to me that epilepsy was one of those disorders for which doctors sometimes could not determine an exact cause. I leaned back in my chair, looked up at the ceiling, took a deep breath, and exhaled slowly. I wasn't going to get the answers I was looking for.

Before leaving his office, Dr. Espy handed me two pamphlets—one called "Epilepsy: You and Your Treatment," the other called "Answering Your Questions About Epilepsy."

WHEN I RETURNED home from Dr. Espy's office, I sat down and picked up the phone to call my parents. Now that I had accepted my diagnosis, it was time to let them know the truth:

I had epilepsy.

CHAPTER 11

OVER THE NEXT few weeks, I poured myself into learning everything I could about epilepsy and seizures and found out that it was a very misunderstood condition. I was shocked to learn that until 1956, people with epilepsy in the US were forbidden to marry in *seventeen* states. I was also surprised to read that epilepsy affected approximately 1 percent of the US population.

I kept reading and learning. The human brain consists of fifty to one hundred billion brain cells and one hundred trillion connections, I discovered. Seizures are like a fire in the brain. All seizures start with a burst of abnormal electricity in the brain; it's like the cells in the brain are communicating too much. Some seizures affect the entire brain immediately, sending it into a frenzy of overactivity. Other seizures start in one specific area but can spread uncontrollably. Their behavior is unpredictable; their duration is unpredictable.

Epilepsy can occur from a brain injury at birth, genetic abnormalities, trauma from a blow to the head, or lasting damage from a stroke or infection. It can spread organically or jump from one brain section to another. But for half of all patients, there are no apparent causes.

And while most people can control their epilepsy with medication, almost one-third of all patients do not respond to their medication, and doctors don't know why.

Reading this, I thought about the one episode I'd had since starting on Tegretol.

Please let me be one of the people who can control their seizures with medication.

CHAPTER 12

A MONTH LATER, I was in a great mood as I drove west down the 10 freeway toward Santa Monica. My buddy Dave—a friend I hadn't seen since moving to LA—was in town from San Francisco, and I was excited to see him.

I'd met Dave during my junior year at St. Mary's College. Dave was also on the baseball team, and we'd instantly hit it off. After graduation, I'd often gone to Dave's apartment in the Haight-Ashbury district in San Francisco, where we'd hang out for a while before going out to hit the clubs and bars. Monday was my favorite night to see Dave, because that meant we would head over to the I-Beam, a gay nightclub in the Haight that hosted a mixed crowd on Monday nights because of the live bands they featured. I saw many bands I never heard of again there, but I also saw some bands that made a name for themselves: The Cure, Duran Duran, The Bangles, Chris Isaak, and the Red Hot Chili Peppers, to name a few. And Dave was the one who had pushed me to apply for a bartending job at the Hard Rock Café in San Francisco in the first place. "You have the look for a Hard Rock bartender," he told me. "You have to try at least." Turned out he was right—and it changed my life in many ways.

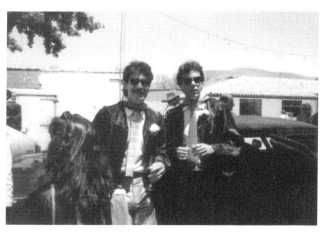

Me and Dave – St Mary's Graduation - 1983

Joining Dave would be his buddy Herman, a guy I hadn't seen since we played baseball against each other in high school. Dave and Herman were in Southern California to play golf in San Diego and visit Dave's brother in LA. They'd just gotten to LA after three days of golf in San Diego, and they wanted to meet me for dinner in Santa Monica.

I knew the perfect place: Gotham Hall.

Gotham was on the Third Street Promenade in Santa Monica, an area the city of Santa Monica had converted into a three-block-long pedestrian mall in the 1960s. They'd redesigned it in 1989, turning it into the Third Street Promenade—which, with more than sixty stores and twenty-five restaurants, cafés, and casual dining spots, was a hot place to be.

Gotham—a pool hall, bar, and restaurant located on the second floor of a converted fraternal lodge—was my favorite place on the Promenade. I thought Prince owned it the first time I walked inside because everything was purple, including the pool tables and couches. But as I walked through the place and noticed the artwork and the snakelike vines on the walls, I quickly realized that the owner of Gotham Hall was paying homage to Batman. It felt like the Joker might walk into the room any second.

I met Dave and Herman in the parking lot and gave them both a big hug before leading them into Gotham. I had made reservations, so we had a table waiting for us next to the bar in the middle of the restaurant.

Dave told me the full story of what happened later, and it went like this:

The three of us were enjoying a drink and a pre-dinner chat when suddenly and without warning, I began to get excited and started tapping the table. I yelled out a few "woo-hoos," and my tapping on the table became stronger and stronger, rattling the place settings enough for Herman and Dave to look at each other quizzically.

My seizure subsided almost as quickly as it began. The server walked over and asked if everything was okay. Dave and Herman answered yes and gave her their order while I straightened the place settings as if nothing had happened. After Dave and Herman had ordered their food, I gave the server my order. Dinner was served and consumed without any further interruptions. Now it was time to rack 'em up and play pool.

After ordering a round of drinks and trying out different pool cues, we decided to play Cutthroat so all three of us could play simultaneously. I racked the balls, and Herman broke. No balls went in any of the pockets, so Dave went next—and missed. It was now my turn.

I slowly walked around the table, always the competitor, looking for my best shot. I then reached down, picked up the nine-ball and placed it near the table's break mark. We were not experts or strict rule followers, but we all knew you could not touch the balls on the table.

I lined up my shot and stared at the nine-ball in front of me.

"What the fuck are you doing?" Dave demanded.

Then it began. I dropped my stick and began clapping my hands and yelling, "Woo-hoo!" I was more vocal and animated than I had been when we were in the restaurant. (With the music blasting in the crowded pool room, my seizure went unnoticed by everyone except Dave and Herman; this was some comfort to me when I heard the story later.)

As I began clapping more rapidly and making my sounds louder, Dave grabbed my left arm. I slapped his hand away like it was nothing, even though he outweighed me by sixty pounds. Then I reached over, grabbed him by the shoulders, and started making a humping movement toward him like a dog in heat. He tried to throw me off him, but he couldn't break my grip.

Then, just as suddenly as I started the bizarre behavior, I stopped: I pulled my hands off Dave, took a step back, and looked at him and Herman with confusion. I knew something had just happened, but wasn't sure what. None of us knew what to say, so we just continued our Cutthroat game as if nothing had happened.

The next day, Herman called me and delicately explained that I had exhibited some peculiar behavior the previous night.

I felt a sinking feeling in my stomach. "What did I do?" I asked.

Dave took the phone from Herman and told me everything that had happened the previous night. When I heard how I'd acted, I felt embarrassed and ashamed that they'd seen me like that—and I knew I had to tell Dave what I was going through.

"I was diagnosed with epilepsy a few months ago," I said. "I've been having these types of seizures since April."

For a long moment, Dave was silent. Then he said, "I am here for you, brother. I love you."

Tears pricked at my eyes. "I love you too." I hung up the phone and lay down on my bed.

I just lay there staring at the ceiling, feeling demoralized. As I looked up at the ceiling, I kept thinking to myself, *Why me . . . why me?*

CHAPTER 13

It was early 1993, and Donnita was excited because her younger sister, Becky, was flying in from Wenatchee, Washington, to see her. She wanted to show her sister the LA nightlife, and she asked if I wanted to join.

Of course, I said yes—and I knew precisely where to take them.

They showed up at my place on Becky's first night in town dressed to kill. Becky wore a black leather miniskirt, a tight white tank-styled bodysuit, and black high-heeled shoes. Donnita, meanwhile, was in the sexiest outfit I have ever seen: a tight black sleeveless minidress with a plunging neckline and black high-heeled shoes.

I suggested we start our outing at Nicky Blair's on Sunset Boulevard to cater to Becky's desire for a glimpse of celebrities. Nicky Blair's was a high-end Italian-style restaurant. The bar was always backed up two deep with locals, young actors, and actresses. You could always count on a Rolls Royce or a Ferrari to be parked in front of the restaurant, and to see some older actors/actresses having dinner there.

Just after we got our drinks, Donnita announced that she had to go to the bathroom. "You want to come with?" she asked, looking at Becky.

"Sure!" Becky said, and off they went while I stayed to babysit our drinks.

They headed through the dining room to the bathrooms, which were located in the back of the restaurant. I noticed men's necks turning as they walked past their tables. I cracked up when I saw two guys sitting at a table with their two dates, and one of the guys elbowed his buddy and motioned with his head to Donnita and Becky as they approached their table. The two guys kept their eyes glued on both women as they walked past their table. I recognized one of them: it was Scott Baio.

After spending an hour at the bar "people watching," we left and went next door to Le Dome, a restaurant/bar that was co-owned by Elton John. It was a remarkably similar crowd to Nicky Blair's. After an hour there, it was time to hit Roxbury.

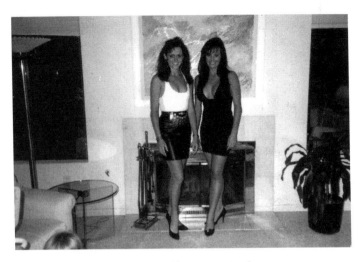

Donnita and her sister Becky

I TOOK BOTH Donnita and Becky by the arm as we walked up Sunset toward Roxbury. As we got closer, Becky noticed the large crowd gathered in front of the club.

"Oh my god," she said, eyes wide. "How are we going to get in?"

"Do not worry," Donnita said cheerfully. "Michael knows the doorman."

The crowd in front of the entrance was about five deep. As we got closer, I started to look for my buddy, the doorman. I saw him and waved to get his attention. He was talking to a group of girls and not looking my way at first, but finally he noticed me.

"How many?" he mouthed.

I held up three fingers.

He whispered into the ear of one of the bouncers, who then pointed to me and waved me over.

I grabbed Donnita's and Becky's hands. "Let's go!"

As we walked through the crowd, the bouncer told people to move to the side. They all stared at us, and I could see them asking each other, "Who is that?"

When we got through the crowd, the doorman walked us into the club. I was pretty sure they didn't have clubs like that one in Wenatchee, Washington. My suspicions were confirmed by the way Becky's jaw dropped as we made our way to the dance floor.

- - -

THE FOLLOWING DAY, Donnita called me to inform me that she had just gotten off the phone with her ex-sister-in-law, Terri. She and Terri were catching up, she said, and then, out of nowhere, Terri said, "My brother (Donnita's estranged husband) called me last night around eleven. He was freaking out."

"What? Why was he freaking out?" Donnita asked.

"He said he was driving down Sunset with his buddy and saw you and another woman arm in arm with this great-looking guy."

"Really? He saw me?"

"Yep," Terri said. "That's what he said. Were you with Michael last night?"

"I was," Donnita responded.

"Good. Because I told my brother he knew the guy you were arm in arm with."

"What?" Donnita was surprised, but also amused. "No, you didn't."

"Yep," Terri said gleefully. "I told him he knew the guy, and he started to freak out and asked me who it was. I told him it was the bartender from the Hard Rock that he said would never give you the time of day."

"You didn't!"

Donnita and Terri enjoyed a good laugh.

"I did!" Terri crowed. "I wish I could have been a fly in that car to see his reaction when I said that."

To this day, Donnita loves to tell people the story about the night I took her and her sister to Roxbury and her ex-husband saw her arm and arm with me—the bartender from the Hard Rock who he said would never give her the time of day.

I love the story too—and I especially love that it was a perfect night, uninterrupted by one of my episodes. It seemed I couldn't count on that to be the case anymore.

CHAPTER 14

MARCH 1993. I had not seen my parents since I was diagnosed with epilepsy. My dad was the pitching coach for St. Ignatius College Prep in San Francisco, and he and my mom were in San Luis Obispo for the weekend for the annual High School Baseball Easter Tournament. I decided to drive up to San Luis Obispo to spend some time with them.

My dad was born and raised in San Francisco and was a standout athlete at Galileo High School. (Galileo has produced some famous sports stars, including O. J. Simpson and Joe DiMaggio.) After graduating from Galileo in 1951, he signed a Minor League contract with the Pittsburgh Pirates. He never made it past Single-A level in the minors, but he did get the opportunity to play with some talented players. One of those was his roommate, Pittsburgh Pirate legend and Hall of Fame third baseman Bill Mazeroski.

In addition to being a coach, my dad was the co-owner of a store on 27th Avenue and Taraval Street in the Sunset District of San Francisco called Flying Goose Sporting Goods. I'd worked there for many years, starting when I was ten.

If you played sports in the San Francisco Bay Area anywhere between the '60s and the '80s, you knew Flying Goose and my dad's name, Tom King. You most likely bought your first baseball glove, your first pair of basketball shoes, your first pair of football cleats, your first pair of baseball spikes, or your high school letterman jacket at Flying Goose. My dad loved baseball, and he loved mentoring kids at all levels: those just learning to play, high school players, and college players. He was also a very generous person. He gave his time, expertise, and resources to young baseball players, never expecting a dime in return. If one of his players needed a bat, glove, or pair of spikes, my dad gave it to them. He would often pull the items directly from the Flying Goose inventory—a habit I am sure his partner at the store did not much care for.

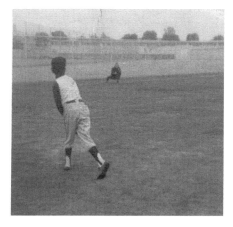

Me pitching to my dad – 1969

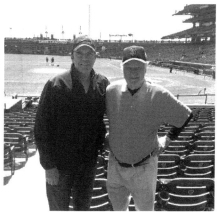

Me and my dad – 2018

My mom was also born in San Francisco and graduated from Balboa High School. She was a fantastic woman who kept everything together in our family. She had a profound sense of style and always dressed in the newest fashions. When my sister and I were little, she always dressed us in adorable outfits as well.

My mom was always there whenever I needed her. When I was young, any time I wanted to work on my pitching, she would grab the catcher's glove and mask and go to the park with me. She was also there for me when I got a bit mischievous. Like in fifth grade when I decided to make an artistic statement with a paper-mache project for school and used pictures from my dad's *Sports Illustrated* and *Playboy* magazines.

One of the most important things my mom taught me when I was young was the value of money. It was about the importance of saving money and how to get deals. She was a great negotiator and made sure I understood the difference between buying something because you "need it" and buying something because you "want it."

In short, my parents were amazing role models who had always had my back. Now, as I faced one of the scariest things I'd ever experienced, it was time to let them be there for me again.

I threw my weekend bag in the back of my car, hopped in the driver's seat, and took off up the coast.

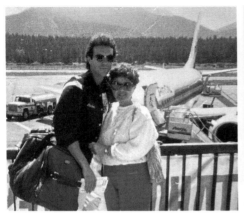 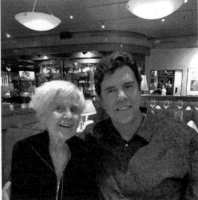

Me and my mom – Lake Tahoe - 1987   Me and my mom - 2021

CHAPTER 15

As I made my way up the 101 freeway, the sun shining on my face and U2's "Mysterious Ways" blasting from my car speakers, I recalled my days pitching for St. Ignatius in the High School Baseball Easter Tournament.

In my junior year, 1977, I was six outs away from beating the mighty Redwood High School—a team that boasted eight future NCAA Division I college players, five High School All-Americans, and six future professional baseball players. (The name that most people remember from that team is Buddy Biancalana, who was the starting shortstop for the Kansas City Royals when they won the 1985 World Series.) Unfortunately, we ended up losing 4–3 to Redwood in nine innings—but considering their lineup, we made a pretty impressive showing.

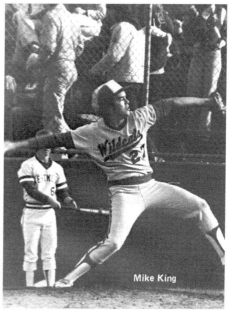

St Ignatius - 1978

After almost beating Redwood in my junior year, I was looking forward to pitching against them in the semifinal game in my senior year. It was about 7:00 p.m. the night before the game, and we had a 10:00 p.m. curfew.

"Let's walk down to the store to grab a snack and something to drink," my best friend John, our starting centerfielder, suggested.

We walked down to the store and picked out some things. While we were at the counter paying for our sodas and bags of chips, three girls entered the store wearing shorts and green-and-white T-shirts. I noticed Cal Poly Mustangs etched on one's shirt. They smiled at John and me as they made their way to the cooler and grabbed two twelve-packs of Budweiser.

We moved off to the side as they approached the counter.

One of the girls looked at me and smiled again. "You want to go to a party?"

"Sure!" we said in unison, and without hesitation we grabbed the two twelve-packs of beer off the counter and jumped in the car with the girls. We were off to our first college party.

Students from Cal Poly filled the house and the backyard. John and I had no idea where we were. We each had a beer and were having a great time when I suddenly remembered our curfew.

I nudged someone near me. "Hey, you got the time?"

He glanced at his wrist. "It's nine forty-five."

I panicked. I raced through the house and the backyard until I finally found the girl that drove us to the party. "You've got to take us back to the hotel," I pleaded. "Like, right now!"

Luckily for us, she agreed. But it felt like it took forever to get back there, and when we pulled into the parking lot, I saw our head coach, Jim Dekker, and my dad standing in front of the door to our room.

As we got out of the car, my dad did not say anything. He just glared at me and shook his head.

Coach Dekker looked at us and said, "Get to bed."

Since we'd missed curfew, John and I had to sit in the stands and watch the game the next day. Our team played a good game but lost to Redwood 5–2.

When we sat down for a team breakfast the following day, my dad walked by and dropped the sports page from the local paper on my plate. He had circled one of the articles. The headline read: *Redwood tries for Easter title.* The third paragraph read, *St. Ignatius was forced to play Redwood without two starters, benched by Coach Jim Dekker for missing curfew Thursday night. One of the two was pitcher Mike King, who earlier had been named to start against the Giants.*

Feeling a little sick, I showed the article to my buddy John.

He just smiled. "I'm glad they didn't mention *my* name."

But it was hard for me to find any humor in the situation. I'd let down my dad, and I'd let myself down too. I hoped I'd never do anything so dumb ever again.

Redwood tries for Easter title

SAN LUIS OBISPO — Redwood of Larkspur goes after its third straight San Luis Obispo Easter baseball title today against Rolling Hills of Los Angeles.

The Giants, behind Jimmy Jones' brilliant one-hitter, subdued St. Ignatius 5-2 in yesterday's semifinal. Rolling Hills eked out a 3-1 triumph over South Torrance to earn its way into today's finals.

St. Ignatius was forced to play Redwood without two starters, who were benched by Coach Jim Dekker for missing curfew Thursday night. One of the two was pitcher Mike King, who earlier had been named to start against the Giants.

Jones gave up only a second inning single to Mike Watkins that drove in one of SI's two runs in that inning.

St. Ignatius meets South Torrance today to decide third place.

Newspaper Article

CHAPTER 16

WHEN I ARRIVED at the hotel in San Luis Obispo where my parents were staying, I parked my car in the lot and headed to their room.

My mom answered the door and gave me a big hug and held on to me tightly, seemingly reluctant to let go.

"How are you doing?" she asked.

"I'm doing okay." I made my way over to the bed and sat down.

She sat across from me in a chair. "How was the drive?"

"It was nice. I stopped in Santa Barbara for lunch." I could tell that something was on her mind. I raised my eyebrows at her. "What?"

"Well . . . did your doctor tell you that it was okay for you to drive?"

"Yeah, I'm fine to drive," I said quickly. "He didn't say I shouldn't be driving. Don't worry."

"It's my job to worry," she shot back. Then she stood up. "Come on, let me show you to your room."

THE NEXT DAY, I watched a baseball game with Mom. After the game, I went down to the field and spoke to my dad and Jim Dekker, who was still head coach of the team. Of course, Mr. Dekker had to bring up the time I broke curfew and couldn't pitch against Redwood. We could laugh about it now.

"Are you joining us for dinner tonight?" Mr. Dekker asked.

The dinner would be a big get-together with the parents of players who'd made the trip, the coaches and their wives, and the athletic director at St. Ignatius, Leo LaRocca.

"I wouldn't miss it," I said with a big smile.

DINNER WAS IN a private room at the restaurant. I sat next to my mom and across from my dad. Some parents knew me from when I played baseball at St. Ignatius, so it was great to catch up with them.

Toward the end of dinner, Leo stood up. "I've got a trick I want to show everyone," he announced. He picked up a bottle of wine and an empty glass. "I can pour wine into this glass while holding this bottle completely upright."

This got a big laugh from everyone at the table. As some parents commented that it was impossible, Leo slowly raised the bottle of wine and the glass.

And that's when, my parents later informed me, I started clapping my hands loudly and shouting, "Woo-hoo!" This continued for about fifteen seconds, at the end of which I turned to my mom and yelled, "I want my keys!"

"I don't have your keys, honey," she said gently.

I continued shouting, "Where are my keys!"

And then, as quickly as it started, it was over.

The room was hushed as I came back to my senses. Things were a little foggy for me, but I knew I'd just had a seizure. I looked across the table at my dad. He just sat there, his eyes fixed on me. This was the first time my parents had seen me during an episode.

People would not look me in the eyes as I looked around the room.

Leo broke the silence by thanking the parents for making the trip out to the tournament and informed everyone that the vans were outside to take everyone back to the hotel.

People slowly got up out of their chairs and headed toward the exit.

I wished I could disappear.

THE FOLLOWING DAY, it was time for me to head back to LA. I gave my mom a big hug and kiss on the cheek. I shook hands with my dad; he was not a hugger.

"Are you okay to drive?" my mom asked.

"Yes," I assured her. "I'm fine."

My mom had to give me one more big hug before she would let me leave. "I love you. Call me when you get back home."

"I love you too. I will."

I got into my car and drove off, feeling sad and ashamed.

CHAPTER 17

AFTER LEAVING HER husband, Donnita had vowed to be on her own for two years. She had been jumping from one long relationship to the next since she was fifteen years old, and now that she'd finally freed herself from her husband's grip, the last thing she wanted to do was jump into another relationship. Even though she'd fallen in love with me, she felt she needed this time to be independent. She wanted to spend time with her friends and not answer to anyone.

I was not thrilled with the idea of her seeing other guys, but she told me it was something she had to do before we could think of having a serious relationship. I told her I would wait for her until I was old and gray. I just kept praying that she would not meet some guy who would be in a position to offer her a lot more than I could—someone who would sweep her off her feet.

Even though I was willing to wait if I had to, I had a crazy idea I might be able to change her mind about dating other guys by writing her a song. I had never written a song before, so I just started writing down things she had shared about her life. Then, one day, a phrase came into my head: *My love is just a step away.* I started repeating the words over and over again, and after a few days, I had a whole song written.

The next time we saw each other, I gave her the song I had written for her. As she read it, tears started to roll down her cheeks. She gave me a big hug. "I love it. Thank you."

I figured now was the time to make my case. "I love *you*. I think that we should just see each other exclusively."

Unfortunately, she did not agree with me. "Let's give it one more year," she said firmly.

A YEAR LATER, I drove down to Newport Beach and took Donnita to dinner at one of our favorite spots in town, Spazzo's. As we sipped our pre-dinner drinks, I silently deliberated how to start the conversation I wanted to have.

Donnita could tell something was on my mind. She looked at me, smiled, and asked, "What's going on?"

I took a big sip of my drink and started: "We both agreed that you shouldn't jump into a relationship with me. We agreed that we should both see other people for two years. Well, it's been two years." I took another sip of my drink and looked right into her eyes. "I do not want to share you with anyone anymore. I would like you to move in with me. Are you ready to do that?"

Donnita was a bit thrown off guard. She looked at me for what seemed like an eternity—then she smiled and said, "Yes, I'm ready."

Just a few months later, in June 1994, she moved in with me.

```
                    MY LOVE IS JUST A STEP AWAY
                         -by Michael King

DEDICATED TO MY LOVE DONNITA

The first time I saw you it was love at first sight
You told me I was too young, it just wouldn't be right
I hoped and prayed that you'd just give me a chance
All I wanted was a try at romance

I know you've been hurt by love before baby but so have I
I know you have your doubts about love, and so do I
Just take this one step baby and you will see
My love for you will set you free...because...

Chorus:
My love is just a step away
Come on baby take that step
Don't be scared and don't hesitate
Because my love is just a step away
I know you're scared baby but it'll be alright
I'll be there for you morning, noon and night
Because my love is just a step away
Come on baby take that step.

My love for you is something that I can't hide
You thought that your love was all locked up inside
When you take that step I'll promise you one thing
I'm gonna unlock all the love that you can bring

Chorus

You've got to believe in love baby
it's a feeling that's next to none
I'm not gonna stop until we finally come together as one

Chorus

When you take that step and take a hold of my hand
I'll promise you I'll be your one and only man
You can forget about the past
because the love I have for you is gonna last and last

Chorus

My love is just a step away, My love is just a step away
Come on baby take that step
Don't be scared and don't hesitate
My love for you is here to stay.
My love is just a step away, My love is just a step away.
Come on baby take that step!

(c) 1993 King Music
All Rights Reserved. Used by Permission.
```

The song I wrote for Donnita

CHAPTER 18

IT HAD BEEN two years since my initial diagnosis of epilepsy, and my sei-zures were starting to happen with more frequency. Donnita told me that I was having at least one seizure a day—and those were just the ones she was witnessing. When I was alone and had a seizure, I wasn't always aware it had happened.

She said that most of them were minor seizures where I would stare at something, softly make odd sounds, and then quickly snap out of it—but I would also regularly have the more severe seizures where I clapped my hands and yelled, "Woo-hoo!"

In July, she and I decided to head to Santa Monica to watch the fire-works to celebrate my birthday. (Yes, my birthday is on the Fourth of July—and it's actually very cool. Everyone has the day off, and there is always a party! When I was little, my mom told me the fireworks were for my birthday. Of course, I had to give my sister a hard time—I always told her it was too bad *she* didn't get fireworks for *her* birthday.)

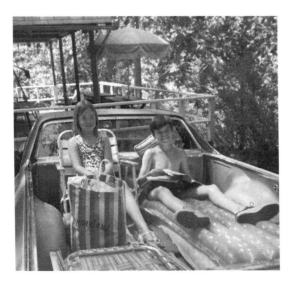

Me and my sister Karen

We found a spot on the crowded beach to watch the fireworks. About halfway through the fireworks show, I started clapping my hands and loudly making sounds. It lasted ten seconds, and then it was over. I looked over at Donnita, smiled, and kissed her. I had no idea what had happened, and Donnita said nothing—not until the next day, anyway.

A WEEK LATER, I had an appointment to see Dr. Espy. I told him about how the frequency of the seizures seemed to be increasing. He decided to increase my carbamazepine (the generic name for Tegretol) medication to 800 milligrams (400 milligrams twice a day). He also wanted me to start taking 200 milligrams of Topamax, an anticonvulsant and nerve pain medication.

As soon as I increased my carbamazepine dosage, I started to feel side effects. I was sluggish; it felt like all the energy in my body had been sucked right out of me. Many days, I just wanted to stay in bed and sleep. Dr. Espy told Donnita that one big seizure was like running a twenty-six-mile marathon.

Since my diagnosis, I'd been trying to figure out what was causing my seizures. Was it flickering lights? That could have been true both at the nightclub and with the fireworks. Was it caffeine? I wasn't a big coffee drinker; I only drank coffee when I wanted a Baileys and coffee. Was I getting enough sleep? Was I eating the wrong type of food?

Nothing I thought of made sense, because sometimes I would have a seizure when I was just sitting at home talking with Donnita.

It was starting to get to me. I just wanted the seizures to stop.

As 1995 STARTED, Dr. Espy decided to take me off Topamax and instead put me on 300 milligrams of Neurontin (another anti-epileptic drug known to help control seizures) once a day and 1,000 milligrams of carbamazepine per day.

Taking these two prescriptions together made me feel even more tired than the Topamax/carbamazepine combo had. I kept hoping Dr. Espy would find the right mix of medicines to control my seizures and not suck all the energy out of my body—but so far nothing seemed to be working out.

CHAPTER 19

IN THE SPRING of 1995, Donnita and I arrived at the Oakland airport for a long-weekend getaway with my parents to Napa. My dad picked us up from the airport and took us back to their house in Concord.

My mom gave me the longest hug when I walked into the house, then stepped back and held my face in her hands. "How are you feeling?"

"I'm feeling good," I lied.

I'd made it a practice to tell my mom about some but not all of the seizures I had. I felt my parents had enough to worry about; I didn't want to add more stress to their lives.

THE NEXT DAY, we made the drive to Napa. It was a beautiful, sunny April morning, and we got up there early.

As we were finishing breakfast, I put down my glass of orange juice and fell into a trance, staring at the salt and pepper shakers in the middle of the table.

My mom called out, "Michael!"

I did not respond.

Donnita touched my shoulder and spoke into my ear, "Michael!"

I did not respond. I just stayed focused on the salt and pepper shakers.

"Grab everything—he's going to have a seizure," my mom called out.

Donnita grabbed the half-full glass of orange juice in front of me just in time; a half second later, I began clapping my hands and yelling, "Woo-hoo!" My mom would later tell me that it felt like an eternity but lasted only about twenty seconds.

After I snapped out of it, I yawned and said, "You guys ready to leave?"

Everyone nodded, so I rose and led the way out, unaware of what had just happened. My parents and Donnita got up from the table and followed me out the door, in silent agreement that no one needed to mention the episode to me.

For the remainder of the weekend, I was seizure-free. It wasn't until we were on the flight home that Donnita told me I'd had a seizure at breakfast.

I did not say anything for the rest of the flight home—I was too angry. Not at her, of course, but at my body, my medication, my situation.

Nothing was working to control my seizures, and I was fed up with all of it.

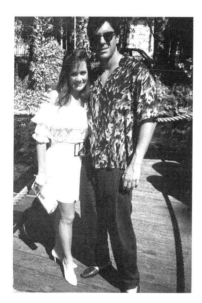 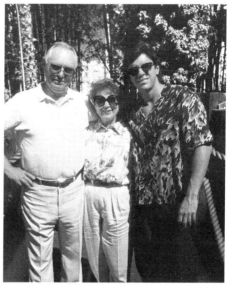

Me and Donnita - Napa   Me and my parents - Napa

CHAPTER 20

As 1996 started, things finally seemed to be calming down with my seizures. Since I was feeling better, Donnita and I hopped in my Nissan 300ZX, popped Alanis Morissette's *Jagged Little Pill* into my tape deck, and headed up 101 to Santa Barbara for a weekend getaway.

Holding Donnita's hand as music played and the sun shone on us, I was the happiest I had been in months.

When we arrived in Santa Barbara, our first stop was Stearns Wharf, where we walked on the pier and took in the views. After that, we stopped by The Harbor Restaurant for an early dinner. It was a beautiful day, so we sat outside.

After dinner, we spent time walking around downtown Santa Barbara. It was a perfect evening—seizure-free.

But the following day, after we got on the road to drive home, Donnita noticed that I was starting to speed up.

"Michael." She tapped my knee. "You might want to slow down."

I did not respond.

"Michael!"

I was now up to seventy miles per hour . . . seventy-five miles per hour. I was beginning to rock back and forth in my seat, and my eyes were focused straight ahead. I was not blinking.

"MICHAEL!"

Again, I didn't answer. Clearly, I was having a seizure.

My hands were positioned at ten and two on the steering wheel. My grip on the steering wheel tightened, and the car slowly started to veer to the left. Donnita grabbed the steering wheel and tugged it toward her, saving us from crashing into the concrete divider.

"MICHAEL!" she screamed again.

But still I did not respond, and I was pushing down even harder on the gas pedal now—we were up to eighty miles per hour.

The car started to drift to the right. The sound of gravel made Donnita grab the steering wheel and return the car into the lane.

I slapped Donnita's hand off the steering wheel.

One strange thing about my seizures was that I could still react to things and even sometimes have a conversation with someone. I just didn't have conscious control of what I was doing or saying and usually didn't remember any of it afterward.

We were now going eighty-five miles per hour.

Donnita reached for the wheel again; again, I slapped her hand away. The speedometer hit ninety miles per hour.

"MICHAEL!" she screamed, tears filling her eyes. she continued screaming my name and started slapping me in the arm, hoping I would come out of it.

Nothing. I continued to rock back and forth in the seat.

Donnita reached for the steering wheel again, and again I slapped her hand away. The car drifted to the left. I was inches from the retaining wall when she managed to grab the wheel and straighten out the car.

One hundred miles per hour.

Donnita frantically leaned in right next to my face and screamed, "MICHAEL!"

Finally, I snapped out of it—and immediately, I realized I was going too fast. I took my foot off the accelerator and braked to slow down. I looked around, trying to figure out where I was. I yawned a huge yawn. Donnita said I always did that after having a severe seizure.

I looked over at Donnita and realized she was sobbing. I had no idea what had just happened, but I could tell from her tear-streaked face that it was not good.

"Pull over!" she yelled as she wiped tears from her face.

Bewildered, I found a safe place to stop the car. As soon as I did, she looked at me and said, "I'm going to drive home."

"Why?" I asked.

"Because you had a seizure while driving!" She was already out of the car and approaching the driver's side. "Get out!"

I slowly opened the door, got out, and walked around the car to the passenger side.

With Donnita in the driver's seat and me in the passenger seat, she pulled back onto the freeway. Within minutes, I was asleep. I slept the entire way home.

WHEN WE GOT HOME, Donnita told me she wanted to talk to me. As soon as we were seated on the futon, she placed her hand on my hand and said, "I don't think that you should be driving anymore. It's not safe."

"That's the first time anything like that has happened," I protested. "I didn't sleep well last night. Maybe that triggered it."

Some part of me knew she was right, but I couldn't imagine not being able to drive. I was trying hard to hold on to the last part of my independence.

"Michael, it's not safe!" she insisted.

"I'll let Dr. Espy know what happened and ask him what he thinks."

"Okay," she agreed reluctantly, and for the moment, she let the subject go.

I did plan to tell Dr. Espy—but not right away. What if I told him the story and he agreed with Donnita?

I decided to hold off on contacting him. *Just for a few weeks*, I told myself.

CHAPTER 21

I COULD NOT keep a bartending job, and I was starting to get incredibly frustrated. I never had a problem getting hired; the problem was keeping the job. And I knew that it had nothing to do with my bartending skills and everything to do with my epilepsy.

I still struggled with whether I should tell a potential employer up front that I had epilepsy. The places where I'd been hired and then fired were starting to add up. Maybe it was time for me to find another job instead of bartending—but what?

Then I received a call from my buddy Michael, who asked if I wanted to work a few nights a week at a new club he was opening on the bottom level of the Beverly Center. The location would be the former site of Ava's and Tramp's. He said he was calling the club Tempest. Of course, I jumped on this opportunity.

"I'd love to," I said excitedly. Then, because I was curious, I asked, "Who else will be bartending at the club?"

He listed the bartenders he'd hired so far. I was familiar with many of them, including Rob Camiletti, Cher's old boyfriend from 1986 to 1989.

I started off working a weekend shift at the club, but the next week I got shifted primarily to weekdays. I learned later that Michael had promised the weekend shifts to the other bartenders to get them to work at Tempest. I needed to find another bartending job for the weekends if I was going to make a living.

While looking over the Classified section of the *LA Times*, I came across an ad Giggles in Glendale had placed, looking for bartenders. When I first saw the name, I thought it was a comedy club, but the ad said it was a two-level nightclub located in downtown Glendale on Brand Boulevard.

Since moving to LA, I hadn't gone into the Valley much. I often stayed on the Westside. But I decided to jump in my car and make the thirty-minute drive to Glendale to check out Giggles and apply for the position.

BE THERE WHEN I RETURN

- - -

As I OPENED the door and entered the club, I was surprised at how big the place was. A man approached me as soon as I walked inside.

"You here to apply for a job?" he asked.

I nodded. "Yes, I'm a bartender."

"Go ahead and fill out an application," he said, handing me a sheet of paper. "My brother will be with you shortly." He held out his hand and said, "My name is Garnick."

I shook his hand. "Michael." He left me alone to fill out the application.

As I waited, I noticed a man who looked like he could be Garnick's brother interviewing another person at a table next to the bar. As soon as the conversation ended, he walked over to me and extended his hand. "Nice to meet you. I'm Edmond."

I gripped his hand firmly in mine. "Nice to meet you too. I'm Michael."

I followed him over to the table near the bar. By the end of our conversation, he'd offered me a bartending job.

I didn't mention the epilepsy.

WHEN I GOT home, I called Michael.

"I was just offered a bartending job at a nightclub in Glendale," I told him. "My shifts will be on Thursday, Friday, and Saturday. Can I work at Tempest every Monday and Tuesday night?"

"Sure," he said. "No problem."

Amazed that everything had turned out so well, I crossed my fingers. Maybe, just maybe, these two bartending jobs would work out and I could stop worrying about how I was going to pay my bills for a while.

By this point, Dr. Espy had increased my carbamazepine dosage to 1,300 milligrams per day and switched me from Neurontin to 350 milligrams of Lamictal per day. The maximum daily dosage is 1,600 milligrams for carbamazepine and 500 milligrams for Lamictal—I was edging toward that ceiling.

What, I wondered, would happen when there was no higher dosage to go to?

CHAPTER 22

On Tuesday, April 30, 1996, Donnita invited me to a small get-to-gether with her Cheesecake Factory coworkers at Valley Park in Hermosa Beach. After playing frisbee and tossing the football for a few hours, it was time for some people, including Donnita, to get to work at The Cheesecake Factory. I also needed to get ready for my shift at Tempest.

I walked Donnita to her car and hugged and kissed her, and she drove off to work. I jumped into my car and started my thirty-minute drive home.

I drove north on Aviation Boulevard, a road with two lanes going in each direction. I stayed in the left lane. The speed limit was forty miles per hour. I knew I had to make a right on West El Segundo Boulevard to get on the 405 North. I stayed in the left lane since it was still a few miles until El Segundo. I looked for Rosecrans Avenue, because El Segundo was the next major street after Rosecrans.

Finally, there it was—Rosecrans. The light was green as I approached the intersection. I looked up for the street sign to double-check the name. Then everything went dark.

The next thing I felt was this strange sensation of being elevated. A few seconds later, I felt like I was moving.

Then I heard a voice saying, "His vitals look good."

I slowly opened my eyes. Things were still very foggy. I looked around, trying to get my bearings. It finally hit me: I was inside an ambulance.

I sat straight up and frantically said, "I need to get my car and get to work!"

"Relax," the paramedic said. "You are not going to be driving that car anytime soon."

A few minutes later, the ambulance arrived at Hawthorne's Robert F. Kennedy Medical Center.

Once in the hospital room, it became evident that I'd had a seizure while driving. The doctor asked me if I remembered what had happened.

"The last thing I remember is crossing Rosecrans," I said. I was wearing a tank top; when I looked down at my arms, I realized they were covered with scratches. I also had a huge knot on my forehead, making me look like Herman Munster from *The Munsters*. I had a cut on my lip and red burn marks across my chest from the seatbelt straps, and my shoulders, jaw, and chin were very sore. I felt like I had gone a few rounds with Mike Tyson.

"You could have sustained much more severe injuries if you had not had a seizure," the doctor said.

I gaped at him. How was that possible?

"If you'd known you were about to crash, you likely would have grabbed the steering wheel to brace yourself and slammed on the brakes, which could have resulted in you breaking your arms and legs," he explained. "Because you were mid-seizure, your body was relaxed, which protected it from greater harm."

Right, but I wouldn't have crashed in the first place if I didn't have epilepsy, I thought bitterly.

Two police officers soon showed up at the hospital to take my statement. I told them exactly what I'd said to the doctor: the last thing I remembered was passing Rosecrans. The officers said that they had spoken to witnesses at the scene and described for me what had happened.

"After crossing Rosecrans, your speed quickly accelerated to sixty miles per hour. You clipped the end of the car in front of you and then veered to your right, crossing over to the right lane, going over the curb, and driving head-on into the trees on the side of the road."

Now all the scratches on my arms made sense.

The officer gave me a hard look. "You are lucky to be alive."

I knew he was right. I sat there for a long time, playing back what had just happened to me and thinking about how differently things could have ended up.

CHAPTER 23

DONNITA AND I arrived at Jim & Jacks Tow in Hermosa Beach two days later to get my car. As I exited Donnita's car and walked toward Jim & Jacks Tow, the paramedic's words—*You are not going to be driving that car anytime soon*—echoed in my ears.

The Jim & Jacks lot was filled with cars with all types of damage, some more severe than others. I looked around for my car, but I couldn't spot it.

"I'll look for it down there," Donnita said, and started to walk down the path that separated the damaged vehicles.

Meanwhile, I spotted someone nearby and flagged him down. "Hey, do you work here?" I asked.

"Yep," he said.

"Any chance you know where my car is? It's a 1984 Nissan 300ZX. It came in two days ago."

"Let's see," he said. "Sounds familiar . . ."

As he tried to remember where my car was located, I looked down the path and saw that Donnita was pointing at something.

"I think my girlfriend found it, thanks!" I said, and jogged down to where Donnita was standing.

The front of the car Donnita was pointing to was facing me—but it was unrecognizable. The front end on the driver's side was bent down and touching the ground. The car's hood was bent in half; I could not see the windshield.

"This is your car," Donnita said.

I just stood there and stared at my car, uncomprehending. *Holy shit! I* thought. *There is no way in hell that is my car.*

But I looked closer—and to my surprise, it was indeed my car. I shook my head in disbelief. Looking at the damage, I realized I must have hit two trees, because the middle and the driver's-side front end were severely damaged, but the front of the passenger side looked untouched.

Donnita took my hand, and we slowly walked around the car together.

The driver's door was slightly ajar, so I grabbed the handle and pulled the door open; it made a loud grinding noise. Then I tried to close the door, but it wouldn't close again. By the look of the damage to the door and the side panel, they'd had to pry the door open to get me out of the car after I crashed into the trees.

I swung the door back open and looked inside. The impact of the crash had pushed the dashboard and steering wheel up toward the windshield. I noticed a crack in the windshield above the steering wheel.

"That's where you must have hit your head," Donnita said.

I reached in and opened the center console and glove compartment and pulled everything out. Then Donnita and I walked around the car one last time. As I took in all the damage, I thought, *The police were right. I am lucky to be alive.*

It finally hit me just how fortunate I was that I hadn't died in the accident—or killed someone else. I started to play the accident back in my mind with a different outcome.

I could have run over a mom walking with her kids on the sidewalk, I realized, horrified by the thought.

Donnita was right. I shouldn't be driving.

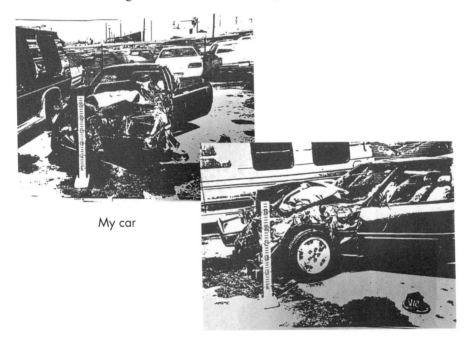

My car

CHAPTER 24

A WEEK AFTER the accident, I met with Dr. Espy and told him about my accident. He thought it would be a good idea for me to go back on Neurontin, but I told him I didn't want to—I really didn't like the side effects. He didn't push it; we agreed that we would keep my medication as it was—1,300 milligrams of carbamazepine and 350 milligrams Lamictal per day.

About a month later, my insurance company informed me that my car was totaled and that I would receive a check for $3,781.28. I also received a letter from the DMV informing me that my driver's license had been suspended since I'd had a seizure while driving.

How was I going to get around LA?

Donnita told me that she would drive me wherever I needed to go, but I felt terrible constantly asking her for rides, so I just started walking to where I needed to go. My doctor's office was about a forty-minute walk, which was not so bad. And when Donnita wasn't working, she could drive me to and from Tempest. The big question was, how would I get to Glendale for my job at Giggles?

After my accident, I spoke to a few bartenders, told them I had car problems—no one at Giggles knew anything about my epilepsy, and I was not ready to share that with anyone—and asked if I could catch a ride home after our shifts together. The big problem was that none of the bartenders lived on the Westside; they all lived in the Valley. Even so, a few said they would give me a ride home after work.

Now I just had to figure out how to get *to* work.

The first thing I did was get a bus schedule and figure out the route to Giggles. It would take me one hour and twenty minutes to get there from my apartment. I decided to leave two hours early to ensure I arrived on time.

ON THE NIGHT of my shift, I left my apartment dressed in my work uniform—black pants and a white tuxedo shirt—and walked one block down

Wilshire to Fairfax. I only had to wait for a few minutes before the bus came. So far, so good!

The sun was setting as the bus drove up Fairfax to Hollywood Boulevard. I knew I had thirty minutes before my next stop, so I sat back and took in all the sights of Hollywood as the bus made its way down Hollywood. I had to get off on North Vermont in East Hollywood, where I would then take another bus that would take me to Glendale.

When the bus driver called out, "Normandie Avenue!" I got up and stretched. North Vermont was just a few stops away.

It was dark outside when I got off at North Vermont and looked around. As I crossed Hollywood and walked up Vermont to the bus stop, I saw drug deals going down and some very shady characters sizing me up. As I approached the bus stop, I decided to stand behind the bus stop bench and lean against a fence so nobody could come up behind me. I made sure I didn't make eye contact with any of the guys who stared at me as they walked past me in the twenty minutes I had to stand there waiting for the bus.

When the bus finally arrived, I climbed inside with relief. It was crowded, but I found a spot in the middle section as the bus made its way up Vermont—and after a few stops, the crowd thinned out. I still had twenty minutes to go before I would get to my destination.

By the time the bus arrived in Glendale, it was only me and two other people on the bus. My stop was coming up. I got off the bus and walked the block and a half to Giggles.

Mission complete.

AROUND 11:00 P.M., Achilles approached my bar with a female friend of his. I'd met Achilles my first night at Giggles, and we'd become instant friends. He was a big sports fan, so we had lots to talk about.

I could not have met the guy at a better time in my life. Six months after I had my first seizure, Tim had left for the US navy. And Rich and Alex never returned my calls again after that night watching the basketball game.

"You want to grab breakfast after your shift?" Achilles asked as I was making drinks for him and his friend.

"I can't," I told him. "My car is in the shop, and I had to take the bus to work." I hadn't told Achilles I had epilepsy yet, and now didn't exactly seem like the right time.

"Wow, the bus? How long did that take?"

I sighed. "About an hour and a half."

"How are you getting back home?"

"Well, that's why I don't think I can do breakfast," I said. "One of the other bartenders said he would give me a ride home."

"Well, if you ever need a ride home, let me know," Achilles offered generously.

And after that first night, he drove me home from Giggles most nights. He was a good friend—someone I could count on. And when he couldn't do it, one of my fellow bartenders always stepped up and helped out.

I'd lost some friends in the last couple of years, but I'd also gained some new ones.

CHAPTER 25

AFTER A MONTH of getting rides home from work, I decided to tell my fellow bartenders—and my bosses—at Giggles that I had epilepsy. I also told Achilles, and made it clear that my car would not be "coming out of the shop" anytime soon. Everybody was very supportive and understanding. I guess you know who your friends are when things get tough.

We had a tremendous bartending crew at Giggles, and we had fun times behind the bar. Besides me, three other bartenders—Kenny, Jeff, and Victoria—were also trying to become actors. Jeff and I had the same agent. Victoria was a background regular on the CBS sitcom *Cybill*, starring Cybill Shepard. The other bartenders were Walter, Stu, and the Nolan brothers, Steve and John. We all got along well.

John in particular always watched out for me when we were behind the bar together. A lawyer by day and a bartender on the weekends, he had been bartending longer than I had and had some remarkable stories. I thought I'd worked at some cool places, but all my stories were nothing compared to John's stories about bartending at the Playboy Mansion.

John, Steve, and I worked at one of the club's main-level bars. I constantly reminded John to watch to see if I started to do something strange. I did not often have seizures at work, but John knew how to handle them when I did. If he noticed that I was starting to have one, he quickly approached me and yelled to the crowd in front of our bar, "Don't worry—he's just messing around." If people kept staring at me, trying to figure out what the hell I was doing, he would stand behind me and hold my arms down until I stopped clapping my hands. Sometimes he made it look like he was holding me and shaking me to the music as it blasted from the speakers—just two friends horsing around. When I had a "small" seizure and just stood there frozen stiff, he'd cover for me until I snapped out of it, and if I forgot what I'd been doing before the seizure hit or how much drinks cost, he'd fill in the blanks for me.

(I did various things over the years to pay John back for taking care of me, the most fun of which was teaching his son, Ryan, how to pitch. Ryan was twelve or thirteen years old and loved to pitch. He had a great arm, and I spent time with him fine-tuning his windup, arm angle, and follow-through. It was the least I could do, after all his dad had done for me!)

I was scared that Edmond and Garnick would fire me for having seizures while on a shift. I decided transparency was my best bet. Any time John told me I'd had a seizure behind the bar, I made sure to tell Edmond and Garnick what had happened at the end of the night. I knew they often saw it as it happened, but I wanted to approach them before they approached me. I always assured them I had never thrown a glass or broken a bottle while bartending. I felt so blessed that Edmond and Garnick knew what I was going through and stood by me during this challenging time.

CHAPTER 26

IT WAS FEBRUARY 1997, and I was bored hanging out at the apartment. Donnita was working, and I wanted to get out of the house and go on a bike ride down to Santa Monica. The problem was, Donnita had freaked out the last time I'd told her I'd gone on a bike ride—"What happens if you have a seizure while you are on your bike?"

So, instead, I decided to go to the Beverly Center and walk around the mall.

I walked down to Wilshire and Fairfax and jumped on the bus. A mile up Fairfax, I got off at Beverly Boulevard and waited for the bus that would take me the rest of the way to the Beverly Center.

Across the street from the bus stop on Beverly was CBS Television Studio. I had been on the lot before, auditioning for CBS soap operas. I noticed a large group of people outside Studio 33; *They must be trying to get into* The Price Is Right, I thought.

I started to get impatient waiting for the bus. I stepped off the curb and looked down Beverly Boulevard to see if the bus was coming. There was no bus in sight.

The next thing I heard was a male voice calling out, "Three dollars!"

I looked around me, confused. *Where the hell am I?* As my senses returned to me, I realized I was in the back seat of a cab, parked in front of the Beverly Center.

I looked at the cab driver.

He shook his head and said—this time with an edge to his voice—"Three dollars!"

I reached into my pocket and pulled out a five-dollar bill. "Keep it," I said as I handed it over.

AS I TOOK the escalator up to the Beverly Center, I tried to play back precisely what had just happened. The last thing I remembered was looking down the street for the bus. I must have had a seizure. *What did I do?*

To this day, I still can't figure out how I waved over a cab and then told the driver to take me to the Beverly Center while I was in the middle of a seizure.

Walking through the Beverly Center, I could not stop thinking about being in the cab. As I walked through the mall, I noticed people looking at me. Over the years, I had become increasingly paranoid when I noticed people looking at me; all I could think was *Did I just have a seizure?* I was never like that before I was diagnosed with epilepsy.

After walking around the mall for about an hour, I decided to head back home. As I made my way down the escalator, I thought about popping into the Hard Rock to see who was working—but decided against it.

Instead of taking the bus home, I decided to walk.

CHAPTER 27

WHEN I ARRIVED back at my apartment, I felt like I had just biked to Santa Monica and back, so I decided to lie down. After sleeping for a few hours, I grabbed my boombox, a folding chair, and two Coronas and headed to the roof to watch the sunset.

Twenty minutes later, I was standing at the edge of the roof—head down, body shaking, tears streaking down my cheeks and falling to the gravel under my feet.

I shut my eyes and whispered a silent plea: *I just want to feel better.*

Then I started to think about my mom and dad. Through all of this, my dad had always told me, "Do not give up. Never give up." And my mom always ended her phone calls by saying, "Be strong. You can beat this!"

They believed in me.

I thought about Donnita too—my rock since I was first diagnosed. I couldn't do this to her. I couldn't do this to any of them.

Tears still rolling down my cheeks, I gently pulled back from the roof's edge—first one foot, then the other. *The medication is not working*, I thought. *There must be other options out there.*

I returned to my chair, sat down, and looked up at the sky as Springsteen's "Better Days" played from my boombox.

I am going to beat this, I told myself. *I am going to beat this.*

CHAPTER 28

A FEW DAYS LATER, the phone rang.

"Hey, Michael, how you doing?"

It was my sister, Karen, calling to check up on me.

I tried to be incredibly positive. I did not tell her about the incident with the cab or what happened on the roof of my apartment. Instead, I asked her how she and my niece and nephews were doing. She then told me the real reason that she was calling:

"I found out recently that someone I know from high school was diagnosed with epilepsy in adulthood, like you, and she had surgery at Stanford Hospital to eliminate her seizures. Do you know about that surgery?"

"No," I said, my mind spinning. "My doctor's never mentioned anything like that."

"Lisa had part of her right temporal lobe removed, and it worked—she doesn't get seizures anymore!"

"Amazing," I said. "I'll definitely look into that!"

Could surgery be an option for me? Was this the cure I'd been hoping for?

Donnita arrived home that evening around six. She walked into the bedroom, looking for me. She called out my name. Nothing. She returned to the kitchen and noticed a note on the refrigerator: *I'M ON THE ROOF – MK.*

She had never gone up to the rooftop with me before. I'd decided to concoct a little surprise for her.

When she made her way to the rooftop and opened the door, I was there waiting for her.

"Surprise!" I yelled out as she just stood there with her mouth open.

Earlier, I'd gone to our favorite Thai restaurant in LA, Chan Dara, and ordered all our usual dishes. I had a large blanket with pillows laid out on the rooftop, facing west. I'd set up two place settings and put a vase filled with flowers in the middle of the blanket. Next to the flowers was a bottle of white wine. I reached over and clicked the Play button on my boombox. Whitney Houston's song from *The Bodyguard*, "I Will Always Love You," began to play.

Donnita's eyes started tearing up as she walked over to me. I hugged and kissed her, and then we sat down on the blanket together.

While we ate, I shared the conversation I'd had with my sister that day. Donnita was just as surprised as I was that there was a surgery that might eliminate seizures.

"Are you going to call Dr. Espy?" she asked.

"First thing in the morning!" I said, grinning.

Years later, I would finally share with Donnita that a few days before our romantic rooftop dinner I'd had my toes hanging over that roof's edge, seriously thinking about ending my life. But that night, I just basked in the excitement we both felt at the possibility I could end my seizures once and for all.

CHAPTER 29

A MONTH LATER, I had an appointment with Dr. Espy. After he asked me how I felt, I told him why I'd made the appointment and asked him if the surgery I'd learned about from my sister was an option for me.

"You could be a candidate for surgery," he said with a nod. "Is that something you would want to look into?"

"Yes!" I said without hesitation. "The medication is not controlling my seizures. I am at the point now that I am willing to try anything to control my seizures."

"Well, if you're really serious about this, you'll need another MRI," he said. "The MRI we did back in 1992 showed no areas of abnormal signal intensity in your brain, but it's possible things have changed since then."

"Fine, no problem," I said. "The sooner, the better."

The results from my new MRI were much different from my 1992 results. This one revealed two small areas on either side of my brain in the sub-Sylvian regions (part of the brain that separates the temporal lobe from the frontal and parietal lobes) with increased signal intensity.

Dr. Espy said he would contact me in a few weeks about possible next steps. I left his office feeling like there was a shimmering of light at the end of the tunnel.

WHEN MAY CAME around, I received the call I was hoping for: Dr. Espy informed me that he'd set up an initial consultation appointment with the epilepsy surgery team at UCLA on Monday, May 12. Donnita and I were over the moon.

Two days before my appointment at UCLA, Donnita and I went to dinner in Pasadena and then to the Pasadena Civic Auditorium to see *A Chorus Line*. I was in a great mood; I decided to spend a few extra bucks and get us seats in the center of the orchestra section.

I held Donnita's hand as the show began.

When it came time for Val's monologue, "Dance: Ten, Looks: Three," the theater was hushed. Suddenly, my left arm started moving up and down, and I began slowly rocking in my chair. Donnita looked at me and noticed that I was staring at a program on the ground beside my foot. I continued to rock back and forth in my chair, my eyes glued to the program.

"Michael," she said softly into my ear.

I did not respond; I just continued to rock back and forth in my chair as I focused on the program on the ground.

She tried again—"Michael!"

No response. I continued to rock back and forth in my chair.

Donnita was nervous and scared. A woman seated in front of Donnita turned around, glared at us, and placed her right index finger in front of her mouth. As I continued to rock back and forth in my chair, a man leaned over my right shoulder and whispered, "Shush!"

Donnita knew what was coming next. I started to clap my hands.

As I began to make my "woo-hoo" sounds, she clamped her hand over my mouth.

A few seconds later, I came out of the seizure. Her hand was still over my mouth; I looked over at her, and her eyes were tearing up. Immediately, I knew what had happened.

I looked around and saw some people looking at me. I sank down low in my seat.

Donnita reached down and held my hand as the show continued. I couldn't wait for that UCLA appointment.

CHAPTER 30

ON MONDAY, MAY 12, Dr. Espy and I arrived at UCLA to meet with the epilepsy surgery team. The team consisted of Dr. Jerome Engel Jr., Sandra Dewar (clinical nurse specialist), and Dr. Paul Mullin, who was doing his fellowship.

Dr. Espy talked a lot as he went through my seizure history from the first time he saw me in 1992, as well as all the medications he'd prescribed me over the years, plus my MRI results.

When Dr. Espy was done, Dr. Engel asked me to describe what I remembered about my seizures. He also asked about my educational history and family medical history; they were very thorough.

As the consultation ended, Dr. Engel told me they would notify me by mail if they felt I was a good candidate for surgery.

THE FIRST WEEK of June, an envelope arrived in the mail from the UCLA Medical Center. I paused momentarily before opening the envelope. *What will I do if they say I am not a candidate for surgery?*

The idea was devastating.

I ripped open the envelope. Inside was a letter from Dr. Engel that said I might be a strong candidate for surgery. He wanted to move me to Phase I of the evaluation process: a PET scan and an EEG. For the EEG, I would be monitored twenty-four hours a day with video recording until I'd had enough seizures for them to document.

This was it—what I'd been waiting for! I ran and showed the letter to Donnita. We were both excited to see if surgery could be an option for me.

ON JUNE 17, I checked into 7 West (telemetry unit of the neurosurgery ward) in the UCLA Medical Center in Westwood. The plan was for me to be in the hospital until the twenty-sixth.

At 8:51 a.m. the next day, June 18, I had my PET (positron emission tomography) scan—a nuclear medicine imaging test they hoped would allow them to locate the part of my brain that was causing my seizures.

The first thing the doctor did was inject me with a radioactive substance called fluorodeoxyglucose (FDG)—a fancy name for simple sugar. Once the FDG reached my brain, they explained, it would send signals read by the scanner, and then the signals would be made into pictures that the doctor would review.

I was then placed on a bed in a dimly lit room and told to remain still for about ninety minutes, long enough for the FDG to pass through my body to my brain. Then it was time for the PET scanner, which looked like a giant donut with a hole in the middle. One of the assistants helped me onto the scanner table and reminded me to remain still as I began to slide into the scanner hole.

After about twenty or thirty minutes, I slid back out of the scanner—it was over.

As I lay in my bed in the Epilepsy Monitoring Unit, I started to think about the next test, the EEG. I kept thinking about the doctor telling me they would slowly take me off my medication and put me on a sleep-deprivation schedule every other day to induce seizures. The idea of having uncontrolled seizures was unnerving. I started to have second thoughts about going through with the EEG.

Then a voice called out from the entrance of my room, "How are you doing, MK?"

A smile came to my face when I saw my good friend George standing there. His timing was perfect.

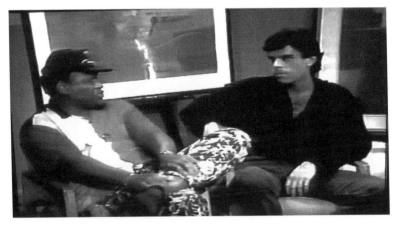

Me and George – Cable Access Show - 1989

George and I had first met in 1987 at a commercial acting class in Studio City. At the time, he'd said that he was a comedian. Everyone in that class wanted to be an actor or comedian, so I thought nothing of it. But after about a week of classes, George asked me if I wanted to hang out with him when he did a set at The Improv on Melrose and then at the Comedy Store on Sunset. Of course, I said yes—and after watching George perform, I quickly realized that he was not just someone *trying* to be a comedian; he *was* a comedian, just like he'd said.

George and I became good friends. I went to a bunch of other clubs with him—Laugh Factory on Sunset, Ice House Comedy Club in Pasadena, The Comedy & Magic Club in Hermosa Beach—and I accompanied him when he appeared on *The Arsenio Hall Show* and *The Keenan Ivory Wayans Show*.

One of our favorite places to hang out for breakfast was Du-Pars on 3rd and Fairfax in LA Farmers Market. As we ate, George would pull out his yellow legal pad of paper and grill me for material—"Did you see anything funny happen at work? Did you hear anyone say anything funny at work? How about at the store?" He was the master of telling "observational jokes." We would sit there for hours and talk about the stupid and/or wild things people said or did.

I had the opportunity to meet a number of other comedians through George—including Jerry Seinfeld, who was his best friend; George was the best man at Jerry's wedding. On a few occasions in 1989, when *The Seinfeld Chronicles* (later changed to just *Seinfeld*) first aired, Jerry joined George and me at Du-Pars for lunch or breakfast. He was usually late, since he refused to park his Porsche in the parking lot (he didn't want a door ding) and always drove around until he could find street parking.

That day at the hospital, George spent about an hour with me in my room. He made me laugh and forget about the EEG—exactly what I needed. During my nine days in the hospital, he visited me three times, and every time it was just when I was feeling down and needed a good laugh. It was like he knew somehow.

When George left my room after visiting that first day, my thoughts immediately returned to the EEG taking place later in the day—but I didn't feel as panicked as before. I was scared, yes, but I knew I needed to have the EEG if I wanted to be considered a candidate for surgery.

And I really wanted that surgery.

CHAPTER 31

IT WAS TIME for my EEG. The technician placed flat metal disc electrodes on my scalp and sphenoidal electrodes, which just looked like skinny wires, into my cheek muscle near my jaw by inserting a thin needle carrying the wire into my cheek and then removing the needle and taping the wire to my skin. (The doctor gave me a local anesthetic to numb the area before they placed the sphenoidal electrodes.) These electrodes would record electrical activity from deep parts of my brain.

After the electrodes were placed, the technician covered my scalp, my forehead, both sides of my face, and under my chin with a white gauze dressing. I looked like I was wearing a big white helmet with a long black cord coming out of my forehead. The technician then connected the EEG transmitter to a wall outlet.

I was then slowly taken off my medication and scheduled to be sleep-deprived every other day. They used a closed-circuit video television to monitor me in bed twenty-four hours a day.

Let the seizures begin!

THE INFORMATION BELOW was taken from the videocassette of my EEG:

June 19, 1997, 3:16 a.m.

I am lying in bed watching a movie. I turn my head to the right. I move my head back to the center. I scrunch my nose and upper lip. I say, "Okay." And then it begins.

I clap my hands together and vocalize, "Woo-hoo!" repeatedly. The entire event lasts approximately ten seconds.

I reach up with my right hand and adjust my glasses (I couldn't wear my contacts during the EEG, so I had to wear my prescription glasses). I have no clue what has just happened.

"Hello, Michael!" a voice booms out from a speaker in the room. It is the technician in the room next door, monitoring my video.

I don't answer her; I just look off to my right.

"Are you okay, Michael?" the technician asks over the speaker.

"Uh-huh," I answer. I am still out of it and don't actually know what she asked me.

I am tired, so I yawn, raise my arms toward the ceiling, and stretch. Then I try to sit up in bed.

My nurse, Sandi, enters my room.

"Was the movie good?" she asks.

"Yeah, it was okay." I shrug. "I've seen it before."

"Did you have a seizure?"

"Did I?"

"Do you know what you just did?" the technician asks through the speaker.

"No. What did I just do?"

"You started to clap your hands and say, 'Woo-hoo!'"

"I did—or I didn't—have a seizure? I don't remember." I'm still not all there.

I try to adjust my glasses from behind my head, but I push them too far forward. As I try to adjust them back into place, my right hand touches the wires coming out of my head.

"Okay—don't pull on the wires, Michael," Sandi says, and reaches up and takes my hand off the wires.

"I am not pulling on the wires. I am just taking them down." I'm still not all there.

VIDEO ENDS – I've just had a complex partial seizure.

June 20, 1997, 3:15 p.m.

Donnita sits on a chair beside me on my right. We are discussing what we want to do for my birthday this year. I am tired. I yawn and cover my mouth with my right hand. We talk about maybe having a BBQ and watching fireworks. Donnita is concerned that she might be unable to get her shift off at The Cheesecake Factory.

I reach to my right and pick up my Day-Timer off my nightstand. I look at my Day-Timer and mention that July 4 is on a Friday. Something catches my attention, and my eyes dart to my right. Then it happens.

I start to mumble unrecognizable words. I yell, "Woo-hoo!" into my Day-Timer. I drop my Day-Timer and it falls to the ground. I begin to clap my hands. I suddenly stop clapping and yelling, "Woo-hoo!"

Sandi is outside my door when it happens, and she hears me clapping and making my sounds. She enters my room and makes her way over to me.

"It's okay, Michael," she says.

"What?" I have no clue what she is talking about.

"What is this?" Sandi holds a pen in front of me.

"What is this?" I repeat what she says. I am still out of it.

"What is this called?" Sandi moves the pen directly in front of me.

I start to mumble some words. I am very frustrated because I do not know what she's holding in her hand. I nervously shift my body around in bed.

"Can you point to the ceiling with your left hand?" she asks.

I raise my left arm and point to the ceiling.

"Can you touch your nose?" she asks.

"With my left or right hand?" I am starting to come out of it.

"With your right hand." Sandi laughs. "You're trying to outsmart me, huh?"

I reach up and touch my nose with my right hand.

"Do you know what day it is?"

"What day is today?" I repeat, trying to figure out what the hell day it is. "Yes?"

I look down. I have no clue what day it is. I finally give it a shot. "It could be Friday."

She nods with approval. I guessed right.

"Do you remember the word that I gave you?" she asks.

I rub my hands together and shake my head no. "What word?"

"Did you hear the word?"

"No."

"How are you feeling right now?"

"I feel fine."

"Who am I? What's my name?"

"You are my nurse." I forget her first name.

"What did you give me yesterday?"

"What did I give you yesterday?" I repeat, again trying to remember.
VIDEO ENDS – I've had another complex partial seizure.

June 21, 1997, 6:34 p.m.

I am watching a baseball game between the Atlanta Braves and Philadelphia Phillies. I feel very relaxed. My hands are on top of the pillow behind my head. After about a minute, I start to lick my lips; then I begin to smack them together. I yank my hands out from behind my head and clap them together in one swift move. I follow that up with a "woo-hoo" sound.

This seizure lasts much longer than the previous two. Sandi walks in and stands next to my bed as I clap my hands and yell, "Woo-hoo!" When I finally stop, I act as if nothing has happened. I calmly adjust the glasses on my face.

"Michael," she says, "can you show me two fingers with your right hand?"

"Can I show you two fingers with my right hand?" Here I go again, repeating what Sandi says to me. I hold up my right hand and show two fingers.

"Where are you?" she asks.

"Where am I?" I have no idea what she's asked me. I hold up my right hand again and show her two fingers.

"Where are you?"

"Where am I?" I start to chuckle, as if she's said something funny. I do not answer her question. I continue to watch my baseball game.

"Can you tell me your name?"

I don't answer her. I adjust the glasses on my face, chuckle, and continue watching the game.

"How many fingers am I holding up?" Sandi holds up two fingers.
"Two."

"What am I holding?" She holds a pen out in front of me.

I don't answer. I just chuckle again, my eyes glued to the TV.

"What do I do with this?" She keeps holding out the pen.

I don't answer her or look at the pen in her hand.

"Can you take this from me and then give it back to me?" She moves the pen closer to me.

I take the pen from her and give it back to her.

"Do you know where you are?"

"The hospital."

"Which one?"

"The main hospital."

"What's the name of the hospital?"

"Umm." I have no clue.

"Is it Cedars-Sinai?"

I shake my head no.

"Is it General Hospital?"

I don't answer her. I continue watching my game.

"Is it UCLA Medical Center?"

"I think so. Yeah."

VIDEO ENDS – I've had another complex partial seizure.

June 25, 1997, 9:38 a.m.

I am now completely off my medication. I am watching TV when something in the room catches my attention and I swivel my head to the left. I reach out with my right hand as if grabbing for something. I stop suddenly. I straighten out my head and prop myself up in my bed.

I reach my hands behind my head and rest them on my pillow. I slide down into the bed, trying to get comfortable. Something gets my attention again. My eyes snap up and to my left. My head shifts to my left too, as if I'm watching a fly make its way through my room. I continue to turn to the left. I release my hands from behind my head as I continue turning my body. I keep turning until I'm almost looking behind me.

I start to slide down the bed. I am now lying on my left side. I begin to make jerking movements. My body stiffens. A deep gurgling sound emerges from my throat. I roll onto my back. My arms stiffen as I raise them toward the ceiling.

I continue to shake as the technician's voice calls out over the speaker, "Michael!"

I do not answer.

My bed starts to make a loud rocking sound as I shake faster and faster. Dr. Mullin and Sandi quickly enter the room. Dr. Mullin moves to the right side of my bed; Sandi moves to the left side of my bed. Dr. Mullin holds me. I shake so vigorously that my glasses are now down by my mouth.

"Take his glasses off!" the technician's voice calls out from the speaker.

Dr. Mullin removes my glasses, then rolls me onto my left side to protect me from choking. I continue to shake and make gurgling sounds that echo through the room.

"Which way are his eyes going?" Dr. Mullin asks Sandi.

"To the left," she answers.

I continue shaking; my body is now as stiff as a board. The muscle spasms are forcing the air out of my lungs. I sound like I am moaning or crying. Dr. Mullin holds me as the shaking finally starts to slow down.

VIDEO ENDS – I've just had a tonic-clonic (grand mal) seizure.

CHAPTER 32

ON JUNE 26, I had another MRI. The scan showed that my ventricles were normal in size, shape, and position. The cerebral sulci (the grooves in my brain) were normal. No masses or bleeding were visible. The signal intensity of my brain was normal in all sequences. The temporal lobes were symmetrical, and there were no apparent abnormalities. The Sab (a crucial signaling platform for neurodegenerative disease) revealed no vascular malformations. My skull was normal, and there was no significant sinus disease. Overall, the impression was that it was a normal MRI.

After monitoring me for nine days, Dr. Mullin and Dr. Engel concluded that I had a syndrome of stereotype complex partial seizures. Based on clinical signs and the EEG, they determined that I had localization-related epilepsy, likely originating in my brain's right central parietal region.

It was impossible to proceed to epilepsy surgery based on the monitoring. Dr. Mullin said he wanted to meet me at the UCLA Medical Center seizure center clinic in three weeks to discuss possibly moving me to a Phase II evaluation, which would entail surgically placing electrodes inside the brain or on the surface of the brain to more accurately establish where the seizures were beginning. In my case, the subdural electrodes would be placed directly on the surface of my brain. This would help them determine where the seizures were located and what part of my brain would be affected if they were to operate, he explained. If my seizures were located in a section of my brain where surgery could potentially damage my memory, speech, and vision, I would not be a candidate for surgery.

Dr. Mullin then recommended that I start taking Dilantin. I had not heard of Dilantin, so I asked Dr. Mullin about its side effects.

"Some possible side effects are headaches, vomiting, loss of balance, slurred speech, dizziness—"

"I don't want to take Dilantin," I said firmly, stopping him there.

"Okay," he said. "In that case, I recommend that you start taking fourteen hundred milligrams of Tegretol XR and increase it to sixteen hundred milligrams after two weeks."

I agreed—and with that, I was discharged from the UCLA Medical Center.

CHAPTER 33

On July 21, I met with Dr. Mullin and Dr. Engel at the UCLA Medical Center. They reviewed my test results again and recommended I move to Phase II. Before that procedure, they wanted me to undergo another MRI, plus a magnetoencephalography (MEG).

The MEG would measure small electrical currents arising inside the neurons of my brain. The combination of images from an MEG and an MRI, they told me, would allow them to more easily locate normal electrical activity in my brain, as well as the areas of my brain that were generating the seizures.

My MRI was scheduled for October 24 at UCLA Medical Center. My MEG was scheduled for October 28 at Scripps Clinic in San Diego.

On October 28, Donnita and I drove to San Diego for my MEG test. My MRI on the twenty-fourth had shown no changes compared to my MRI on June 26. But this MEG test, a new one for me, would hopefully show us something we hadn't seen yet.

EEG electrodes were glued all around my head, and then one was placed over my heart. Three small coils were glued to my forehead, and two other coils were attached to earplugs. I lay down on the MEG bed, where a small metal coil touched all the different dots around my head to record its shape. The information would go into the computer.

After the technician had recorded my head shape on the computer, it was time for the MEG. The sensors were put over my head but did not cover my face. The coils and EEG electrodes were plugged into the sensors. The technician told me that she would be leaving the room. Before she left, she showed me where a small microphone was located so I could talk to her if I needed something.

Like the MRI and PET scan, I had to remain as still as possible, not moving my head. They'd told me the MEG test would take between one and two and a half hours. It felt like it took forever.

A FEW WEEKS later, I received a call from Dr. Mullin. He told me they'd reviewed all my tests and would like me to return to UCLA on December 15 and start Phase II of the evaluation.

"You should expect to be in the hospital until the first week of January," he said. "We'll send you more information in the mail."

"Okay," I said—half-excited to be moving to Phase II, half-scared about them cutting open my scalp and placing electrodes directly on my brain.

Stay positive, I reminded myself. This might be my only path to surgery and becoming seizure-free. No matter what, I had to follow through.

After telling Donnita the excellent news, I called my parents to give them the news. My parents were thrilled that I was moving on to Phase II.

"We want to come out and be with you while you're in the hospital," my mom said.

I could tell she wasn't going to take no for an answer.

"Dr. Mullins mentioned that UCLA has a hotel called Tiverton House that accommodates relatives of patients in the hospital," I said. "It's only five minutes from the hospital. Do you want me to book you guys a room there?"

"That sounds perfect," my mom said.

After we hung up, I called the Tiverton House and booked a room from December 14 to January 9. It was comforting to know that my parents would be nearby.

ON SATURDAY NIGHT, December 13, I bartended at Giggles—my last shift before going into the hospital. At the end of the night, as the entire staff was having our after-shift drink, Edmond presented me with a card signed by everyone, wishing me the best of luck with the surgery.

I felt myself tearing up as I read the card. It was touching to know that the people I worked with genuinely cared about me. I hadn't had that feeling for a long time.

I left for home that night feeling resolved. It was time to go to UCLA and get my epilepsy under control.

CHAPTER 34

THE NEXT DAY, Donnita drove me to the UCLA Medical Center. Once I was settled in, I called my parents and gave them my room number. They told me they would come over that night to have dinner in my room. In the meantime, Donnita was there to keep me company.

About an hour later, Dr. Mullin, Dr. Engel, Dr. Itzak Fried, Nurse Sandi, a psychologist, and a radiologist entered my room. They went over what I should expect during my time in the hospital. Dr. Fried would be the one to surgically place subdural electrodes in the shape of grids and strips on the surface of my brain.

"We plan to do the surgery tomorrow," Dr. Engel finished. "Do you two have any questions?"

"What are the risks of having this type of surgery?" Donnita asked him.

Days earlier, Donnita and I had read over all the literature from UCLA about the procedure and the possible risks, so we already knew the answer to this question—but she wanted to hear it from Dr. Engel.

"The most common risks are possible bleeding and maybe some headaches," he said.

She and I looked at each other, and I nodded.

I looked back at my doctors. "I am ready to do this," I said.

The team told me they would see me tomorrow and left my room.

WHEN MY PARENTS arrived that evening, they each gave Donnita a big hug and then walked over to me. My mom gave me a big hug and a kiss; my dad, as usual, shook my hand.

"How are you doing?" my mom asked.

"Great!" I said—and I meant it. I was excited to see if I was a candidate for surgery. I smiled. "What's for dinner?"

"Italian!" my mom said cheerfully, clearly happy to see me in such good spirits.

They'd brought lasagna and salad from a local Italian restaurant for dinner. It was delicious, and we had a lovely evening catching up.

Before they left, my dad checked in with me. "Are you nervous about the surgery?"

"I'm just trying to stay optimistic that everything will work out," I said. "It has to, right?"

"Right," he said.

Having Donnita and my parents by my side gave me the comforting reassurance I needed to get through the next few weeks.

THE FOLLOWING DAY, the anesthesiologist was the first person to visit me. After thoroughly reviewing my medical records, he informed me that the right side and the top of my head would need to be shaved as part of the procedure.

"Will I be awake during surgery?" I asked.

"No," he said. "I will put you out once we are in the operating room."

Strangely, I was not nervous about being out during the surgery. I was at a point where I was just excited to get this surgery going.

When it was time for me to go to the operating room, Donnita gave me a big hug and kiss and said she loved me. I told her I loved her too and assured her everything would be fine.

Her eyes filled up with tears.

"Everything will be fine," I whispered in her ear, and gave her another kiss. I had to remain positive. I was smiling as they wheeled me out of the room.

HERE'S HOW MY SURGERY WENT, according to my medical records:

Once I was out, a catheter was inserted. Compression stockings and pulsating sleeves were applied to my legs to prevent blood clotting. I was then placed into a full lateral position, with my left side down and my shoulders hanging over the edge of the bed. My left arm rested comfortably on a cushion. In this position, all the pressure points were well padded. My head was stabilized in a three-point fixation and pointed an additional thirty degrees toward the floor. My head was shaved, prepped, and draped. Now it was time for the incision.

Dr. Fried carefully made a horseshoe incision over my right transverse sinus, the part of the brain that allows blood to drain from the back of the head; it includes the anterior occipital (rear part of the upper brain), the posterior parietal (upper back part of the brain), and the posterior temporal region (bottom middle portion of the brain, just behind the temple).

The scalp flap was then secured using fishhooks. Moist gauze was placed over my scalp. Dr. Fried placed three burr holes—holes in the skull used to help relieve pressure on the brain when fluid, such as blood, builds up and starts to compress brain tissue—about one centimeter above the transverse sinus and placed additional burr holes in the parietal and posterior temporal region.

Dr. Fried performed a craniotomy using a Midas Rex drill; the bone flap was elevated off the dura (the tough outer layer of tissue covering and protecting the brain and spinal cord) and placed in gauze for the duration of the surgery.

Dr. Fried now directed his attention to the dura. He placed sutures to elevate the dura, then opened the dura using a scalpel and secured the dural flap over my sinus. The outermost layer of my brain was carefully inspected and found to be normal.

Next, Dr. Fried carried out electrocorticography in the confines of the craniotomy as well as under the bone. The electrocorticography (ECoG), a type of monitoring that uses electrodes placed directly on the exposed surface of the brain to record electrical activity from the cerebral cortex, showed some active spiking, mainly in the anterior extent of the craniotomy over three rows of the electrode grid. Dr. Fried conducted the ECoG several times while he adjusted the grid on my brain.

A forty-eight-contact grid was placed in the final position to encompass the active area of my brain, which showed spiking (fast waves in my brain activity). Dr. Fried then placed one subdural strip under the dura to reach the anterior temporal region, along with a few small two-by-five and two-by-six strips under the bone. Finally, he placed a small four-contact strip in the right parietal region.

When all this was done, he performed evoked potentials (EP) tests to measure the time it took for my nerves to respond to stimulation. There are several types of responses; Dr. Fried used a somatosensory response.

This is when an electrical pulse stimulates the nerves of the arms and the legs.

Stimulation was performed on the contralateral median nerve on my wrist. Dr. Fried spent an hour using several sets of recording sites. The recordings were made from the strip of electrodes placed directly over my brain's cortex. The areas of early negative and positive peaks were identified as my hand's sensory and motor regions. There were no significant complications in my testing.

With all electrodes now in place, the dura was closed using sutures. The bone was then laid back into position using three mini plates. The electrode cables were channeled through a separate incision in my scalp and secured with sutures and anchoring sutures.

The wound was irrigated with bacitracin, a small drain was left in the subgaleal space (the loose tissue space in the scalp), and my scalp was closed with sutures. My scalp was then secured to the skin with staples. The wound was dressed with Polysporin, Xeroform, dry gauze, and Kerlix.

I was released from the three-point position, extubated, and taken to the ICU.

CHAPTER 35

AFTER RECOVERING IN the ICU, I was moved to the Epilepsy Unit, where a technician connected the electrode cables to equipment that would continuously record my brain activity. Later that day, Dr. Fried and Dr. Mullin came into my room.

"The surgery went well," Dr. Fried said. "We'll be monitoring your brain activity for the next six days; after that, we'll look at the data and decide on our next steps."

Over the next six days, I relaxed in my room with my parents and Donnita. Achilles came to visit me in the hospital, and George came a few times too. My spirits were high.

After six days of monitoring, Dr. Mullin and Dr. Engel entered my room to discuss the results. We all crossed our fingers that I would be moving to the final phase: surgery.

"Your seizure pattern is actually quite complex," Dr. Engel said. "After looking over the data, we've concluded that your seizures might be emanating from the mesial parietal, the posterior cingulate area, or perhaps from the mesial temporal area."

Those were three totally different parts of my brain. I looked over at Donnita with a blank look and then mouthed, "What?"

How is it possible that they have no idea where my seizures are coming from?

"So, what does that mean?" My mom looked at both Dr. Engel and Dr. Mullin for answers.

Dr. Engel paused. "We will need to go back in and place additional subdural strips."

"What? Another surgery?" I could not even look at the doctors; I was so mad.

"Yes," he said—apologetically but firmly.

I looked over at Donnita. I could not believe what I had just heard.

The doctors could tell I was upset. "Why don't we give you a moment?"

Dr. Engel suggested. "We'll come back in an hour, and we can talk some more about this."

After I calmed down, I talked to my parents and Donnita. We agreed that I should have the second surgery if it meant that they could precisely locate my seizures.

When the doctors returned to my room, I told them I wanted to have the surgery to add the additional subdural strips.

ON DECEMBER 23, I was wheeled into the operating room for a second time. Like my first surgery, I was placed on the operating table with my face upward and given anesthesia, and shortly after that, I was out.

This time, Dr. Fried inserted two eight-contact subdural strips and one twelve-contact strip. Everything went smoothly, and when he was done, they took me back to the ICU, hopeful that this time we'd be able to get the information we needed.

WHEN I FINALLY got back to my room in the epilepsy unit, Donnita was in my room and could tell I was not in a good mood. I been trying to stay positive, but being in the hospital and having two surgeries was starting to weigh on me.

"Don't worry, baby." She kissed me on the cheek. "Everything is going to work out."

"I still cannot believe that I had to have two surgeries for them to locate my seizures," I complained. "I hope I didn't just undergo two seven-hour surgeries for nothing."

"You need to stay positive," she said. "Everything is going to work out."

"I sure hope so." I lay down in my bed and looked up at the ceiling.

The electrode cables were connected to the wall, and monitoring started again.

CHAPTER 36

A DOCTOR ENTERED my room the next day carrying a small computer console. He asked me how I was feeling and told me he was there to do some testing with the electrodes connected to my brain. He disconnected the electrode cables from the wall unit and attached them to the computer console. He explained that he would stimulate the electrodes to map the functional areas of my brain. I got out of my bed and sat in a chair. The doctor told me to relax, and the testing began.

The doctor pushed a button on the console to stimulate a section of the electrodes. Nothing happened. He pushed a different button on the console, and suddenly, the fingers on my left hand started to move. I looked down at my fingers and tried to stop them from moving, but I couldn't. He pushed the button again, and my fingers stopped moving.

I looked at him, frowning. "That was bizarre."

He pushed another button, and I started to giggle. He pushed the button again and I stopped.

"Recline the chair so your feet are off the ground," he said.

I reclined my chair. He pushed another button. Suddenly, my left foot started to move back and forth. He pushed the button again and my foot stopped moving.

During the testing, I kept thinking back to a day in my high school biology class when we'd placed electrodes on a frog and watched it jump. It was pretty disconcerting to be the frog.

CHRISTMAS DAY WAS approaching, and Donnita had the great idea of having Christmas dinner in my room. When my mom and dad called in the morning to check on me, she spoke to my mom and laid out her plans for Christmas dinner. As soon as we hung up with my parents, I had Donnita call Achilles to see if he could join us that evening too. To my delight, he was immediately on board.

At 6:00 p.m. on Christmas Day, a fantastic aroma filled my room.

Donnita and my parents had come straight from Ralph's supermarket with a premade turkey dinner (turkey, mashed potatoes, stuffing, baked yam casserole, cranberry sauce, rolls) and an apple pie. Donnita had also thought to get plates, glasses, and silverware—everything we needed for a memorable Christmas dinner. Sitting in my room with her, my parents, and Achilles, I almost forgot that I was in a hospital, had just undergone two brain surgeries, and had another possible surgery in the next five days.

My room smelled so good that people walking down the hallway kept trying to figure out where the incredible aroma was coming from. A few staff members stopped in front of my room and looked in, and were surprised to see us enjoying a full turkey dinner with plates, glasses, and silverware. Nurses stopped by my room and peeked in. I invited them to join us, and a few did. As I enjoyed a piece of apple pie and ice cream, I felt confident that the doctors could locate my seizure activity.

ON FRIDAY, DECEMBER 26, Dr. Mullin came into my room to check on me and let me know that I was scheduled for an MRI the next day. "And in two days, on Sunday, we'll be gathering the data from your monitoring," he reminded me.

I crossed my fingers.

MY MRI THE NEXT DAY showed mild right cerebral hemispheric swelling—no focal edema (fluid buildup), no parenchymal (functional tissue in the brain) bleeding, or infarction (obstruction of blood supply). A small extra-axial fluid collection (fluid within the skull but outside the brain tissue) was present beneath the craniotomy flap. Besides that, the doctors said, everything looked good.

LATER THAT DAY, I had a visitor I was excited to see: my buddy Dave. The last time I'd seen him was when we'd gone to Gotham in Santa Monica and I'd started humping him. This time, Dave was in LA for a business meeting and wanted to come by and see me.

Dave smiled as he walked into the room and gave Donnita a hug—but his face fell as he walked over to me. I don't think he'd expected me to look the way I did: my head wrapped in bandages, wires coming out of my head and connecting to a wall unit. It was a lot to take in.

But Dave recovered from his shock, and he spent about an hour with me. He told Donnita about some of the crazy things we did in college and after college, and he asked me how the testing had been going and if surgery was still an option.

"I'll know more in the next few days," I told him.

I was getting tired; Dave noticed. "Well," he said, rising from his seat, "it's time for me to go. I love you, brother. Stay strong." He gave me a big hug.

"I'm trying," I said, returning the hug. "I love you too."

I was glad Dave stopped by to see me, but the moment he was gone, my thoughts turned to what my doctors would tell me the next day. Would I be a candidate for surgery? Or had all this been for nothing?

CHAPTER 37

THE NEXT DAY—SUNDAY, DECEMBER 28—Dr. Engel, Dr. Mullin, and Dr. Fried entered my room to discuss their monitoring findings. Donnita and my parents were in the room with me.

Dr. Engel explained that monitoring and testing showed activity in my brain's right temporal and parietal regions. He also let us know there was a broader activity region in the right parietal region than my right temporal region. Since that was the case, he said they wanted to discuss a type of surgery called a multiple subpial transection (MST). The surgery would only be performed on the right parietal region of my brain. He also said I might need additional surgery on the right temporal region, but they wanted to start with the region with greater activity (my right parietal).

"What, exactly, is an MST?" I asked Dr. Engel.

The only type of epilepsy surgery I had heard of involved removing the section of your brain that was causing the seizures. Were they going to cut out a chunk of my brain?

"The fibers in your brain that are needed for function (speech, sensation, movement, and memory) are arranged vertically within the brain tissue," Dr. Engel explained. "But the fibers that spread seizure activity are arranged horizontally. During an MST, we make a series of shallow cuts, interrupting the horizontal fibers but not the vertical fibers. This allows us to prevent the spread of seizures while preserving the brain's critical functions."

I had already undergone two surgeries, so I was ready to get this done. I nodded, satisfied with his answer.

My mom, however, had another question for the doctor: "What are the risks involved with this type of surgery?"

"Like any surgery, blood clots, infection, or stroke are risks," he said matter-of-factly. "The possible complications with this type of surgery could be swelling in the brain and damage to healthy brain tissue. There could also be short-term and long-term memory loss or trouble speaking some words. And with this type of surgery or any other surgery, there is no guarantee that Michael will not have seizures again."

Donnita didn't want to hear that. I looked over at Donnita, whose eyes were full of tears. She lowered her head and took a deep breath. She wiped her eyes. I grabbed her hand and kissed it. It was a lot for all of us to take in—but for some reason, I wasn't worried about the possible complications from this surgery. This was my one chance to be seizure-free. If I suffered some memory loss as a result—short-term or long-term—I was okay with that.

A hush had fallen over the room. Sitting there, a funny thought came to my head. (During a tense moment, sometimes everyone needs a good laugh!)

"Can I ask you a question, Dr. Engel?" I asked.

"Sure. What?"

"If I gave you some dates, could you erase them from my memory during surgery? There are some events in my life that I definitely want to forget about."

Donnita looked up at me and just shook her head. My dad had a confused look on his face—*Did you just say that?* My mom, who always got my sense of humor, chuckled.

Dr. Engel just shook his head and smiled.

"Let us give you some time to talk about the surgery," Dr. Fried chimed in. "We will be back in an hour."

After the doctors left my room, there was not much to discuss. My mom reiterated the possible complications Dr. Engel had mentioned, but I was in the same place as before: I wanted to have the surgery. I was willing to try anything to be seizure-free. My parents and Donnita stood behind my decision.

So, when Dr. Mullin returned an hour later, I told him I was ready to proceed with the surgery.

He handed me paperwork that needed to be completed before the surgery. "I'll schedule your surgery for Tuesday the thirtieth."

"Sounds good," I said, already starting to fill out the paperwork.

THAT EVENING, I had dinner with Donnita and my parents in my room and watched TV. I was in a good mood; I remained very optimistic about having a successful surgery.

But after they all left to let me get some rest and the night went on, my positive thoughts turned a little dark, and I started to think to myself, *What if?* What if I ended up having short-term and/or long-term memory loss? What if I still had seizures after the surgery? What if this was a big waste of my time and money? What if I didn't remember who Donnita and my parents were when I returned from surgery?

I did not sleep much that night.

CHAPTER 38

It was the early morning of December 30—time for my surgery. I went through the same initial prep as my two previous surgeries.

Once Dr. Fried had exposed the full extent of the region of my brain requiring MST, he took a small biopsy from a region in the anterior-middle part that was active on the ECoG, where electrical stimulation had not elicited a functional response during mapping, and then—under microscopic magnification and illumination—he started the subpial transections.

The transections (cuts) were about five millimeters from each other. Small pieces of Gelfoam were used to control the bleeding.

Once Dr. Fried completed his transections on the planned area, his team performed an ECoG. It showed a significantly changed ECoG, without the previous abnormalities. However, there were still some infrequent spikes in the craniotomy's mid and anterior parts, so he decided to perform more transections. After this second round of cuts, the team performed another ECoG and found the record had been even further improved.

Dr. Fried now moved on to the cortical surface of my brain. Further flushing showed points of cortical bleeding. The wound was flushed with sterile saline solution, and all the subdural electrodes were removed. The removal was done by cutting the cable inside the wound and then pulling the cables from inside to outside.

The dura was closed with sutures. The bleeding in the epidural compartment was stopped by cauterizing and applying Gelfoam. The bone was then placed back into position and secured with mini plates, and the burr holes were covered. To cover the bony defect, a small titanium mesh cranioplasty was placed over the craniectomy region. The wound was then flushed again with bacitracin. My scalp was closed with sutures and then secured to my skin with fifty-eight staples. The wound was dressed.

I was then released from the three-point fixation, extubated, and taken to the neurologic intensive care unit for observation overnight.

CHAPTER 39

As I lay in the neurologic intensive care unit, immersed in a realm between consciousness and slumber, a voice pierced through the surrounding silence, calling out my name—"Michael."

Gradually, I blinked my eyes open, allowing the hazy fog of sleep to dissipate. As my vision cleared, I looked upward and saw three figures standing by my side, their features blurred.

I heard my name called again—"Michael!"

Recognition hit; my eyes widened, and the world around me gradually came into focus. It dawned on me that it was indeed Donnita who had called out my name. I reached out for her hand and interlocked our fingers. Gently, I brought her hand toward my lips and kissed it. Tears welled up in her eyes.

I locked eyes with my parents and saw tears glistening in their eyes as well. I responded with a smile, assuring them that everything was okay, before I closed my eyes and fell back asleep.

The doctor's words about the possibility of short-term memory loss had profoundly impacted Donnita and my parents. Donnita told me later that the moment I reached up, took her hand, and kissed it, she knew I remembered her.

On December 31 at 2:00 p.m., I was returned to my room from the neurologic intensive care unit. When I arrived, my parents and Donnita were there waiting for me. I was still exhausted, I had a bit of a headache, and my right jaw was sore, but I was excited to see my parents and Donnita and hugely relieved that I still knew who they were.

My eyes felt heavy, and my mouth was parched. I spent most of the day sleeping. During this time, my parents and Donnita had the opportunity to meet with Dr. Fried, Dr. Engel, and Dr. Mullin and thank them for taking care of me.

THE NEXT DAY, January 1, I was in good spirits when my parents and Donnita arrived at my room. My headache and sore jaw had subsided, and I was regaining some energy. After a few hours, my mom and Donnita left, and my dad and I watched Michigan and Washington State duke it out at the Rose Bowl. What a way to start the new year.

My mom and Donnita returned later with Chinese food from Chin Chin on Sunset. My mom always ordered too much food; she thought I would have a bigger appetite. We ended up giving the leftovers to the nurses.

OVER THE NEXT few days, the doctors were surprised by how quickly I was recovering. I was on a regular diet and could walk through the hospital without much assistance.

The first time I went on a walk after my surgery, as I was making my way out the door with my nurse, I heard Donnita call out, "Nice butt!"

I looked back and she gave me a wink.

Why can't they design a better hospital gown? I wondered, even as I chuckled.

ON JANUARY 3, my nurse Sandi entered my room carrying a folder full of papers.

I was getting anxious to go home, so I hoped she was there to deliver some good news.

"How are you feeling?" she asked.

"Fine. I feel really good."

"Let me take a look at your head." She made her way around to the side of my bed and looked at the horseshoe-shaped staple design on my head. "It looks like it's healing nicely."

A nurse had come into my room earlier in the day and removed the gauze from my head. By the look on Donnita's face as this happened, she'd had no idea how large the incision was and how many staples had been needed to close the incision until that moment. After the nurse left, she'd helped me into the bathroom so I could look at the incision for myself. When I got the angle of the small mirror in my hand right and was able to see my reflection properly, the look I'd seen on Donnita's face had made sense; I looked like a patient of Dr. Frankenstein.

After checking my head, Sandi pulled a paper from her folder and reviewed her checklist. I passed her tests, so she signed off that I was okay to be released from the hospital. "Go ahead and fill out these release papers," she told me, handing them over. "You'll be released tomorrow morning."

Donnita and I were both excited to hear that news.

"Thank you for taking good care of him," she told Sandi.

"You're welcome. He was a good patient." Sandi smiled at me.

"Thank you, and thank you for taking care of me," I said.

"My pleasure." She gave my hand a squeeze, then turned and left my room.

ON SUNDAY, JANUARY 4, Dr. Mullin visited my room and reviewed the medications he wanted me to start taking: 500 milligrams of Tegretol XR three times a day, and 20 milligrams each of Decadron Taper and Pepcid three times a day. "And we'll have you come in on January twelfth to get those staples removed," he added.

"Thank you for everything," I said, shaking his hand.

"You are welcome." He then directed his attention to Donnita. "Please let me know if he has any complications or seizures before I see him on the twelfth, okay?"

"I will, and thank you again for taking care of him." Donnita hugged Dr. Mullin with tears in her eyes.

A nurse entered my room with my two-wheeled limousine. I said one last goodbye to Dr. Mullin, and then we were out the door and heading down the hall, Donnita following close behind.

It was time to go home.

CHAPTER 40

IT WAS GREAT to be back in our apartment. The first thing I did after we arrived was walk into the bedroom, put my bag down, and lie spread-eagle on our bed, face up. It was great to be back in a real bed after being confined to a tiny hospital bed for the last three weeks.

After I lay there for a few minutes, Donnita and I walked down to the pool and jacuzzi. I was looking forward to getting back into the water.

When we returned to our apartment, I was tired and decided to take a nap.

The next thing I knew, Donnita was calling my name.

I looked up and saw her seated next to me on the bed. Confused, I tried to process where I was. "Did I have a seizure?" I asked.

"Yes," she said.

"What did I do?"

"You started shaking your head. You started to shake your head so fast that your lips were flapping. Then you started snorting like a pig."

I rolled over in bed so my back was now facing Donnita. After everything I'd gone through, I was right back to having seizures?

"Remember what Dr. Mullin said? That there was a chance that you would have a seizure—that it's normal for that to happen after surgery?" Donnita rubbed my shoulder.

"Yeah . . . I know," I said softly.

That knowledge didn't make me feel any better about the fact that I had seizures throughout the day and night—four total—my first day home. They were all unlike my typical seizures; instead of clapping my hands and yelling, "Woo-hoo!" I shook my head so hard that my lips flapped. And almost every time, I made a different sound—sometimes a snort, sometimes a gurgling sound, sometimes a high-pitched sound like I was trying to say *help*. And through it all, Donnita was always by my side, ensuring that nothing bad happened to me.

Had I undergone three surgeries for nothing?

Donnita continued to remind me that Dr. Mullin had said it was normal for me to have seizures after surgery. I tried to stay positive, but it was tough. When she was with me, it was easier to stay positive, but when she left to go to work and I was by myself, I started to go to dark places: *What if the surgery was unsuccessful? What if I continue to have seizures? Is that a life worth living?*

CHAPTER 41

THE FOLLOWING DAY, I called Dr. Mullin and told him about the seizures. He assured me it was normal and there was nothing to worry about. He decided to increase my daily Tegretol XR intake by 200 milligrams, which got me up to 1,700 milligrams of Tegretol per day.

A few days after my call with Dr. Mullin, my right arm began tingling, and then the fingers on my right arm followed suit. I wasn't sure what was happening. Donnita wasn't home. I waited a few minutes, and the tingling sensation didn't disappear. Did this have anything to do with my brain surgery?

I grabbed the phone, called the UCLA Medical Center, and spoke to one of the nurses. She told me that the tingling in my arm was part of the brain's healing process after surgery. "It should go away soon," she told me. "But if it doesn't, call back, okay?"

"Okay," I said, a bit uncertainly. "Will you let Dr. Mullin know that I called?"

"Of course," she said.

Only slightly reassured, I hung up the phone. But she was right—just a few minutes later, the tingling sensation in my right arm went away, never to return.

AFTER BEING STUCK in a hospital and now my apartment for weeks, I wanted to get outside, walk around, and feel the sun on my face.

"I'm going stir-crazy," I told Donnita. "You want to walk over to the museum with me?"

"I don't think you're ready for that yet," she said, shaking her head.

"Please," I pleaded. "I have to get some fresh air."

"Well, it is less than half a mile away . . ." She thought for a moment. "Okay. Let's do it."

I grabbed my San Francisco Giants hat to cover my nasty scar, and off we went.

Everything went smoothly, and I felt great after our short walk. But Donnita worried I was pushing it too hard. "You just had multiple brain surgeries," she reminded me. "You have to let your body rest more!"

Of course, I did not agree with her. "I feel fine," I insisted. "You worry too much!"

LATER THAT NIGHT, we had Chinese food from Chin Chin. As we were finishing dinner, Donnita opened up her fortune cookie—and started giggling.

"I think this one was meant for you," she said, and handed it to me.

TAKE IT EASY! it said.

We both had a good laugh.

"Okay . . . okay," I relented. "I will take it easy until my next appointment."

"Thank you," Donnita said with a sigh of relief.

CHAPTER 42

DONNITA AND I ARRIVED at UCLA Medical Center three weeks later to meet with Dr. Mullin. This was an exciting day; I was getting the fifty-eight staples in my head removed.

"How are you feeling?" Dr. Mullin asked as we shook hands.

"I feel good," I said.

"Have you had any seizures since I increased your medication?"

"Just the one small one two days after you increased my medication."

He looked over at Donnita. "That's the only one?"

"Yes," she confirmed.

"Have you experienced the tingling in your arms and fingers again?" he asked as he positioned himself to the side of the examination table.

I shook my head. "No."

"Good. Now, let me take a look at your incision."

I took off my baseball hat, and he examined the incision thoroughly. "It looks good," he said with a nod of approval. Let's get those staples out."

He wiped down my incision with rubbing alcohol and started removing the staples with a pair of small surgical pliers. There was a slight pinch and tug every time he removed a staple, but it was not that painful. Every time he took out a staple, though, I noticed Donnita cringing as if she were having the staples removed from her own head.

"Don't worry," I said, "it really doesn't hurt!"

When Dr. Mullin finished removing the last staple, he wiped down my incision one final time. "Everything looks good!"

"So what's next?" I asked.

"When you come in on February third, Dr. Engel and I will assess your progress since the surgery and discuss if you need another MST," he said. "Until then, take good care of yourself!"

"I will," I said. *And I really hope I don't need another surgery*, I added silently.

CHAPTER 43

A MONTH HAD passed since my surgery, and it was time for my follow-up appointment with Dr. Mullin and Dr. Engel. As Donnita drove us down Wilshire Boulevard, she glanced at me in the passenger seat. My body was shifted to the right, and I was leaning on my shoulder, so my back was turned to her. I stared out the window at passing cars.

"What's going on?" she asked.

"Just thinking."

"About what?"

"About what happens if they tell me I need to return for another surgery." I shuddered. "I don't know if I can go through that again."

"Try to think positive," she said. "You have had only one small seizure since Dr. Mullin increased your medication."

"I know. I know. I'm trying."

It's just hard.

AT THE APPOINTMENT that day, Dr. Mullin checked to see how my scar was healing—everything looked good—and Dr. Engel checked my blood levels and asked me about my memory.

"Well, about a week ago we had a friend over at our apartment, and they were talking about when we all saw Elton John at the Hollywood Bowl in 1995," I told him. "I don't remember ever seeing Elton John at the Hollywood Bowl."

"Are there any other events you don't remember?"

"None that I'm aware of," I answered honestly.

"When was the last time you had a seizure?" Dr. Engel asked.

"I had one small one after Dr. Mullin increased my medication," I said. "That was back on January eighth. I have not had a seizure since then. I feel great."

"Good," Dr. Engel said. "If you continue to be seizure-free, there is a good chance that you will not need a second surgery."

I almost jumped off the exam table with joy when I heard that. I was not looking forward to another operation.

Dr. Mullin decided to take me off Decadron Taper and Pepcid but keep my Tegretol XR medication the same—1,700 milligrams daily.

Donnita and I crossed our fingers.

CHAPTER 44

A WEEK AFTER my follow-up examination at UCLA, Achilles picked me up and, at my request, took me to the Glendale Galleria Shopping Center.

The whole way there, he kept asking me why I needed to go to the Galleria.

"I'll tell you when we get there," I said, and refused to say any more.

By the time we entered the Galleria, I could tell the suspense was killing him.

"Follow me," I said mischievously, and led him through the shopping center.

"Where are we going?" he pleaded.

I stopped in front of a store. "Here!"

Achilles looked up at the sign: CLASSIC DESIGN JEWELRY. He gave me a quizzical look.

"I want to ask Donnita to marry me," I said, grinning.

"Amazing!" he said, returning the grin. "Well, let's go buy a ring!"

As we looked over rings with the salesperson, I thought about what type of ring I wanted and described it to him. He showed me a few rings—none of which were what I was looking for.

Finally, frustrated, I asked him for a piece of paper and a pen. I am not the greatest artist, but I was able to draw what I wanted: a ring with a diamond in the middle and smaller diamonds around the larger center diamond.

"I think I have exactly what you're looking for," he said, and led me straight over to a ring with small diamonds circling an empty center. "You'll have to pick a diamond for the center yourself," he explained.

He placed individual diamonds on the counter, and I picked out a one-carat diamond. The ring would be eighteen-karat yellow gold with the diamond I'd just selected in the center and six marquise-cut diamonds surrounding it. It was perfect! I knew paying off the ring would take a while, but Donnita was worth it.

"It will be ready on Saturday," the salesperson said once we'd finalized the paperwork.

Achilles clapped me on the back as we left the store. "So, when are you going to pop the question?"

"Sunday night!" I said with a tremor of excitement.

I couldn't wait.

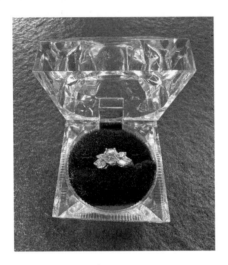

The Ring

CHAPTER 45

THAT SUNDAY EVENING, I walked into The Arches restaurant with Donnita; Donnita's best friend, Gigi; and Gigi's husband, Bob. The Arches had been a staple in Newport Beach since the early 1920s. It was your classic restaurant, with big red leather booths and white tablecloths. Bob and Gigi were in on the surprise, of course. They'd promised to help me make it a perfect evening.

I nervously played with the engagement ring in my right pants pocket as we walked to our table. I kept thinking back to standing on the rooftop, feeling so hopeless, and then thinking about where I was now—looking forward to the future, about to ask Donnita to marry me. I had a hard time believing that this was actually happening.

As always, Donnita looked beautiful. She wore a stunning sheer leopard-print turtleneck top with a black miniskirt. I was wearing black pants, a black shirt, and a black jacket and was rocking my newly purchased black beret, perfect for covering my half-shaven head and scar.

We sat down at our table and ordered a round of drinks. While we waited for them to arrive, Gigi leaned over to Donnita. "I need to go to the bathroom—come with?"

"Sure!" Donnita slid out of the booth.

As the two women walked to the bathroom, Bob waved the server over to our table.

Bob and Gigi were regulars at Arches. Bob had spoken to the manager before we arrived to let him know that I was going to propose to Donnita and wanted the server to place the ring in her dessert.

I pulled out the ring and handed it to the server. "Here you go. Thank you."

The server left the table, and the girls returned a few minutes later from the bathroom.

We had a leisurely, delicious meal. Finally, the plates were cleared from the table, and it was time for dessert. The server approached the table.

"Would the ladies care for some dessert?"

"We'll have a cheesecake to share," Gigi said, gesturing to Bob.

The server turned his attention to Donnita. "What would you like for dessert?"

"Nothing, thank you," she said. "I'm full."

The server looked at me, confused.

I turned to Donnita. "Come on, let's split a dessert."

"No," she said. "I'm full. If you want something, get it."

Gigi gave it a shot. "They have the best cheesecake, Donnita."

Donnita finally gave in. "Okay. I'll have a scoop of vanilla ice cream."

The server looked at me again, now very confused. He was probably thinking, *Am I supposed to put the ring in a scoop of ice cream?*

"I'll have a piece of cheesecake," I said quickly.

As the server left the table, I worried what Donnita might be thinking. Had we ruined the surprise by pushing her to have cheesecake?

A few minutes later, the server arrived at our table with two plates of cheesecake and a bowl of vanilla ice cream. He placed the first cheesecake in between Bob and Gigi, with two forks. Then he moved over to Donnita and, looking at me, placed the cheesecake in front of her. And there was the ring—right on top of the whipped cream in the middle of the cheesecake.

"No, I ordered the vanilla ice cream," Donnita said, sounding vaguely annoyed. Then she looked down at the piece of cheesecake and noticed the diamond ring in the whipped cream. She looked over at Gigi. Gigi smiled. She looked at me. I nervously cracked a small smile. She looked up at the server and said, "I guess I'm having the cheesecake after all."

With that, tears of joy filled her eyes, and she gave Gigi a big hug.

"Well, are you going to say yes?" Bob asked cheerfully.

Donnita turned and looked at me, her eyes shining.

"Will you marry me?" I asked.

"Yes!" she cried out.

"I wanted to ask you to marry me a few years ago," I said softly, "but I thought you deserved a healthy man."

I'd felt Donnita might be "the one" since the first time we met. But the issues I'd been dealing with for the last handful of years had made me feel like I would never be in a position to ask her to marry me. She had always been there for me, though, and now it was official—we were getting married! She'd said YES!

I reached over, took the ring from the cake, and wiped off the whipped cream, then placed the ring on her finger. People clapped and yelled congratulations as we hugged and kissed.

After dessert, we left the restaurant and drove to Bob and Gigi's house, where we enjoyed a glass of champagne and took tons of pictures.

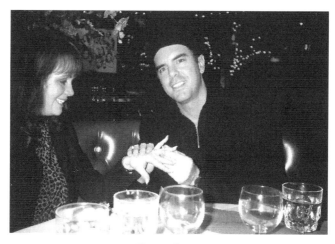

She said yes!

Less than a month later, on March 3, I received a bill from UCLA Medical Center for Phase I testing totaling $23,697.57. I gaped at the number, my heart in my throat.

If that's just for Phase I, I immediately thought, *what will the bill for the Phase II testing and the surgery look like?*

CHAPTER 46

EVEN BEFORE MY SURGERY, Donnita and I had discussed having a baby—but we were of course worried about my epilepsy. What would happen if I had a seizure while feeding or holding the baby? During one of my earlier appointments with Dr. Mullin, Donnita had mentioned that we wanted to have a baby, and he'd said it was quite rare for a parent to pass epilepsy down to their child. But he'd also said that the reproductive rates for men with epilepsy were lower versus women with epilepsy, which had stuck with me. Was I even capable of having a baby?

A few weeks after I asked Donnita to marry me, she came home from work and pulled out a small soapstone elephant figure. "Jackie gave it to me," she said. "It's from India—she says she's given it to a few of her other friends, and all of them have babies now. Worth a try, right?" She placed the elephant on her nightstand.

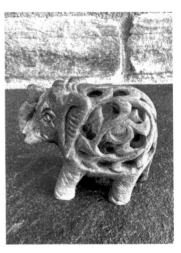

The soapstone elephant

Anything was worth a try, as far as I was concerned.

THREE MONTHS LATER, Donnita didn't feel right. The night before, we'd gone into Westwood and had dinner at an Italian restaurant called Mario's. She thought she might have food poisoning, or at least had eaten something that had disagreed with her.

I went to the store for groceries and left her home alone. She felt awful and didn't know what to do, so she called her mom.

When Donnita described her stomach pains and nausea to her mom, her mom didn't skip a beat. "You're pregnant," she said calmly.

That thought had never crossed Donnita's mind. We'd been trying, but she had assumed it would take us longer to get pregnant—more like a year, not just a few months.

"Go get a test," her mom said, totally sure of herself.

Donnita drove the two blocks to Rite Aid and picked up two pregnancy tests, along with a Pepsi.

Once back home, she was nervous but excited to see the results. She went into the bathroom and pulled out the first test kit. She urinated on the test stick and sat down to wait the three minutes until the results would show. While waiting, she twisted off the top of her Pepsi and took a sip. Pepsi was running a campaign where you could win money and prizes with a specially marked plastic twist-off cap at the time, so Donnita looked under the cap—and was stunned to see that the word printed there was BABY.

The timer went off. Donnita picked up the stick, almost afraid to look at the results.

Just then, I returned from the store and walked into the bedroom. I saw Donnita standing in the bathroom, holding something in her hand, but I couldn't tell what it was.

"What is going on?" I asked.

Donnita thrust the pregnancy test in my direction. "I'm pregnant!"

I stood there frozen for a minute, not knowing what to do or say.

Donnita grabbed the box that the test came in and handed it to me. "Here, read the directions to make sure."

I read the directions, and they were clear—no room for error. I shook my head with disbelief. "You are pregnant."

She grabbed the second test she'd bought and opened it. "I want to retake it to make sure."

We waited together, and when the timer went off, we found that the second test had come out the same as the first.

By this point, I'd had enough time to recover from my initial shock and start to feel excited. Donnita was pregnant, just as we'd hoped.

I hugged her and kissed her. "We are having a *baby!*"

CHAPTER 47

WE STARTED TALKING about what our life would be like with a baby, now that it was really happening. How could we care for an infant with us both working at night? Donnita was currently bartending four to five nights a week at The Cheesecake Factory in Redondo Beach, and I was back to working four to five nights a week between Giggles and Tempest. It quickly became apparent that one of us had to find a day job.

As we discussed how to make this work, my dad's voice kept entering my thoughts: *Get a college degree—you never know when you'll need it!*

Good thing I'd listened to him.

"I'll start looking for a job," I told Donnita. "I'll figure something out."

Now the big question was, *What the hell do I want to do?*

Since graduating from St. Mary's, I had only worked as a bartender. I didn't even know where to start. But I would figure it out.

DURING THE FOLLOWING MONTHS, I diligently scoured the Classified section of the *LA Times* every day in search of a job. The biggest problem was that I did not know what I wanted to do. I interviewed at restaurants as a daytime manager and for some entry-level sales jobs, but I knew that wasn't where my passion lay. It was easy for me to see when something was wrong for me; I just wasn't sure what might be *right*.

After weeks of failed attempts to find something that felt like a good fit, I became very frustrated, so I took a break and decided to dust off my golf clubs.

The last time I'd played golf had been when I still worked at the Hard Rock in LA. Back then I'd play at least twice and sometimes three times a week with guys I worked with: Michael Linehan, John O'Donnell (OD), Paul Medhurst, Marc Poppel, and Calvin Vaughn. We played Griffith Park (Wilson & Harding), Rancho Park, Industry Hills, Balboa Golf Club, DeBell Golf Club, Los Verdes Golf Course, and Malibu Golf Club. I missed playing, but I had lost touch with the guys over the years, so I didn't really have anyone to go with anymore.

Until I met Kevin.

I'd gotten to know Kevin, who DJ'd on Thursday nights (Country Night) at Giggles, over the last few months. We had talked about playing golf some weekend, and on a Thursday night in early September, he finally suggested a specific plan.

"Want to play this Saturday morning at ten?" he asked as I made drinks behind the bar.

"Sounds great!" I said. And it did—great to get back on the course, and great to do something besides job hunt on a Saturday. I was in.

KEVIN SWUNG BY my place on Saturday morning. I tossed my clubs in the back of his car, and we headed down 6th Street. Only then did I realize, *I never asked him where we were playing.*

"So, where are we playing?" I asked.

"I made a tee time at Harding," he said.

"Really?"

Kevin could tell by the tone of my voice I was not thrilled with his choice. "You don't like Harding?"

Griffith Park is a vast park—the second-largest park in California, in fact—located in the Los Feliz neighborhood of Los Angeles. It boasts two eighteen-hole courses, Harding and Wilson, which are always booked from sunrise to sunset on the weekend.

"It took over five hours the last time I played that course," I said with a groan. "You couldn't get a time anywhere else?"

"We could probably get on at Balboa if you want to head out to Encino," he said.

"No, that's fine," I said quickly. I didn't want to go that far. "Harding it is."

WHEN WE ARRIVED at Harding, Kevin and I walked into the pro shop and paid our green fees. As we walked toward the exit, the door swung open. I grabbed the door and held it open for three guys who were coming into the shop. To my surprise, I recognized the last guy to walk in.

"Calvin!" I said.

He turned and his eyes widened. "Michael!"

He and I hadn't seen each other since 1989. I gave him a big hug.

I looked at Kevin and said, "This is Calvin. We bartended together at the Hard Rock, and he was one of the guys I used to play golf with all the time. Calvin, this is Kevin."

Kevin and Calvin shook hands. "I'll grab a cart and meet you outside," Kevin said with a wave, and he walked out the door.

I was excited to see Calvin. "So, what are you doing nowadays? Are you still bartending?"

"No more bartending for me," he said with a laugh.

"Cool—what are you doing now?" I asked.

"I'm a recruiter."

I paused for a second. I had not known anyone who worked as a recruiter before. "A recruiter?" I repeated. "So, do you recruit for the army or the navy?"

Calvin chuckled. "No. I recruit for software companies in Silicon Valley."

He pointed to the two guys he'd walked in with, who were now at the counter paying the green and cart rental fees. Calvin told me that they owned the recruiting company, and two other guys worked at the company as recruiters like him.

The only thing that came to mind to ask next was "So, are you making good money?"

Calvin smiled. "I should be able to make a hundred thousand dollars this year."

I would love to make $100,000 a year, I thought. As I fantasized about what it would be like to make that much money, Calvin's bosses walked back over to us.

"Michael, this is Rick and Craig," Calvin introduced us.

We shook hands and exchanged pleasantries, then moved toward the shop exit together.

"What time are you guys teeing off?" I asked.

"At ten fifteen," Calvin said.

So, they would be playing behind us. "You want to grab a drink after the round?"

He glanced at Rick and Craig, and they nodded yes. "Sure!" he said.

"Awesome, see you guys after, then." I looked forward to catching up with Calvin some more. And I had a lot of questions about this recruiting thing.

THAT AFTERNOON, we all sat down and shared some appetizers and a few pitchers of beer. I couldn't stop thinking about Calvin's $100,000 salary, and I wanted to learn more about the job. I asked Rick and Craig to tell me about their company.

Rick did most of the talking. "It's called Littler Savage, after our last names," he said, then explained their history and what they did.

Rick was closer to my age. Craig was fifteen to twenty years older than me, but he was a good-looking guy for his age. I would later find out that he was an actor who'd appeared in *Blazing Saddles*, *Days of Our Lives*, and *Dallas* and played Jason in the series *Jason of Star Command*. He'd also been the guy in the 1981 Grey Poupon commercial who pulled up in the back seat of a Rolls Royce and asked, "Pardon me, would you have any Grey Poupon?"

As we were wrapping up our drinks, Craig looked at me and said, "You should come down to the office in Santa Monica and see what we do."

It was exactly what I was hoping to hear. "I would love to," I said. "I'm free Monday morning, if that works for you guys."

Craig looked at Rick, and Rick looked at me. "Why don't you come by at ten o'clock that morning?" he suggested.

"I'll be there!" I said.

As Kevin and I walked out the door and headed to his car, all I could think was *Good thing I didn't talk Kevin out of playing golf at Griffith Park!*

CHAPTER 48

ON MONDAY MORNING, I embarked on the fifty-minute bus journey down Wilshire Boulevard, heading to 4th Street in Santa Monica.

When I got off the bus, I walked straight to 322 Santa Monica Boulevard, entered the building, and looked at the directory on the wall. There it was: LITTLER SAVAGE. I took the elevator to the third floor and entered the office.

As I entered the office, Rick was seated in the corner, typing away on his computer. His attire—shorts and a vibrant Hawaiian shirt—surprised me. I'd expected a more formal environment, so I'd worn khaki dress pants and a white dress shirt.

"Michael!" Rick rose from his desk, smiling, and crossed over to shake hands with me. "Let me give you the tour," he said.

There was a long table in the middle of the room with two computers and stacks of papers. The space was tiny. He walked me into an adjacent office, where I saw Calvin at his desk on the phone and two more desks near him with guys seated at them, also busy on the phone. Craig was seated at a fourth desk in the back left corner of the office. Rick headed to Craig's desk, and I followed.

"Hey, Michael, how are you?" Craig got up to shake my hand, and immediately I noticed that he was also dressed very casually. I felt a bit overdressed and awkward, like I should have known better. But there was lots of energy in the office, and I loved it.

Rick and Craig and I chatted for a few minutes.

"I should probably get back to work here," Craig said after a bit, "but why don't you go and sit with Calvin for a while—get an idea of what the job entails?"

"Sounds great!" I said.

Calvin said hi and introduced me to the other two recruiters. All three guys were wearing shorts and either a T-shirt or a short-sleeved shirt. If I didn't know any better, I would have thought they were recruiting people to work for surfing or swimwear companies instead of tech companies in Silicon Valley.

I grabbed a chair and sat across from Calvin's desk. As I sat down, the first thing I noticed was that Calvin's wall next to him was covered with yellow Post-its, divided into two separate sections. "What are those for?" I asked.

He pointed to the first section. "These are people who are interviewing with some of our clients." He pointed to the other section. "These are people I need to find roles for."

My gaze shifted to a large stack of white papers on his desk. "And what's that?" I asked.

He picked up the stack and flipped through it. "This is an employee phone directory for a software company in the East Bay called Sybase. Rick buys the employee directories from a third party and splits them between us. We call every person in the directory to see if they are interested in looking for a new job. If we don't get them on the phone, we leave a message and email them."

"How do you know their phone number and email?" I asked.

"When we call, we just dial the main office and ask for the person."

"And their email?"

He pointed to the top of the page, where *firstinitiallastname @sybase. com* was written in pen. "Rick gives us the company email format," he explained, "and then we send them an email."

"Do you know what job they do at the company when you call them?"

"Nope. We have a bunch of different roles we work on, so I just try to get someone on the phone, and then I find out what they do at the company."

"You guys don't use those job boards like Dice, HotJobs, or Career-Builder?"

"Nope." Calvin shrugged. "Rick said they have been considering trying one of them, but we only have the employee directories right now."

I still wasn't clear on what Rick's and Craig's roles were. "Do Rick and Craig also call people all day?"

"No, they manage the clients," Calvin explained. "They get the jobs from software companies in the Bay Area, and we find the candidates to fill the roles."

I sat there for the next two hours and watched Calvin make one call after another. Most of the time he just got people's voice mail and ended up leaving a message, but sometimes someone did pick up the phone. When that happened, I listened as Calvin read from a script on his desk. He introduced himself and said a few words about what Littler Savage did, then asked the person what they did at Sybase and if they were open to hearing about something new. If the person said they were not looking to make a move, he looked down at his script and read the "response for a candidate not looking" back to the person. Some of these calls were quick (sometimes people even hung up on him), but some lasted a while and sounded like good conversations. Over the two hours I watched him work, Calvin found ten people open to hearing about something new.

On the piece of paper he was reading from, I noticed that he had written, *LOCATION: HOME PHONE NUMBER: CELL NUMBER (IF THEY HAVE ONE): PERSONAL EMAIL.* "Why do you need that information?" I asked.

"Where they live is important because we have clients all over the Bay Area—San Francisco, East Bay, Peninsula, and South Bay," he said. "They're sometimes more open to changing jobs if we have a client with an office closer to their house, so that's good info to know. And Rick and Craig always want us to try to get their personal email, home number, and cell number if they have one so we can get them in the database and keep track of them."

Now it was time to send emails. I followed Calvin into the adjoining office, where the two computers the recruiters used were located. I sat next to Calvin as he pulled up a template to email the people at Sybase with whom he'd left voice messages. The email was just like his voice message: he introduced himself, told them about Littler Savage, and mentioned the different roles he was working on (engineering, business development, marketing, tech support, QA, professional services, and sales). He ended the email by asking them to get back to him if they were open to hearing about something new.

After sending those emails, he moved on to the ten people he'd talked to who'd said they were interested in hearing more. He pulled up a template that asked them to send him their résumé and explained that he would get back to them with companies and roles that would fit their background once he reviewed their résumé.

"I have to show Rick and Craig their résumé before I tell them anything," he told me. "They're the ones who decide if the person has the right background for a specific company and role."

I watched Calvin send out email after email. As I watched him tick off another name on the list, I finally voiced the question I had been dying to ask him: "So, how do you get paid?"

"I get paid when Rick or Craig places one of my candidates at one of their clients," he said. "They bill the company twenty percent of the candidate's first-year base salary, and the payment terms are net 30, so the check usually arrives thirty to forty-five days after the person starts. I get thirty percent of the amount paid, and the average salary for the roles we work on is a hundred thousand, so I make around six thousand dollars per placement. My goal is to make at least two placements a month."

Since this was all new to me, I continued with the questions. "Do you have to set up all the interviews and talk to the company about how much they will pay the person?"

"Nope." He grinned. "The only thing we do is find the candidates. Rick and Craig do everything else."

As I sat there thinking about how nice it would be to make $12,000 a month, a voice called out, "Lunchtime! Let's go down to the Promenade."

AFTER LUNCH, I returned to the office with the guys, and Rick and Craig asked me to walk back with them to Craig's desk.

"So, what do you think about what we're doing here?" Rick asked.

"It's great!" I said enthusiastically. "I think I could be a good recruiter. I love talking to people. And I noticed that Calvin has a giant map of the Bay Area on his wall so he can figure out how far people live from the companies he's recruiting for . . . Since I grew up in the Bay Area, I won't need one of those! I know the area well."

"Well, we don't have an open desk right at this time," Rick said.

All my excitement about being a recruiter quickly vanished.

"But," he said, lowering his voice, "we might have one in three months."

Apparently one of the recruiters was struggling, and Rick and Craig didn't think he'd last much longer. But since they were all friends, they'd given him three months to catch up. If he hadn't billed a specific number by the end of that period, he would be done.

"Check back with us in two months," Craig said.

I shook hands with Rick and Craig, said bye to Calvin, and left the office feeling disappointed that they hadn't offered me a job on the spot but still hopeful that I might get a chance to be a recruiter.

I walked back to Wilshire Boulevard, jumped on a bus, and headed home. Two months wasn't so very long, after all.

CHAPTER 49

WHEN NOVEMBER ROLLED AROUND, I had been seizure-free for almost ten months—since January 13. My medication was still the same: 1,700 milligrams of Tegretol XR per day.

Since first being diagnosed with epilepsy and prescribed medication, I had been very diligent in taking my medication, and Dr. Mullin continued to remind me every time we spoke of the importance of taking my medication at the correct dosage and at the correct times. Everything was going so well that I was starting to feel that my surgery might have worked after all.

Just a few days into November, I received a call from Rick at Littler Savage. The call was very short: Rick said, "You want to give it a shot?" and I responded with an emphatic "Yes!"

After hanging up with Rick, I ran into the bedroom to tell Donnita the good news. Unfortunately, when I explained the terms of the job—100 percent commission, no benefits, and I would be on a 1099, so I would have to pay my own taxes—she was not as excited about it as I was.

I understood her concerns and admitted I was having the same thoughts. I decided to keep my bartending job at Giggles until I knew for sure this new gig would work out. Meanwhile, Donnita would continue to work her four shifts a week at The Cheesecake Factory while she was pregnant. Once the baby came, and she went back to work, she would only work night shifts Monday through Thursday and occasionally on Sunday.

I really hoped being a recruiter would work out so I could quit my bartending job once and for all.

CHAPTER 50

MY FIRST DAY AT Littler Savage was one week later. I wore dress pants and a dress shirt again, even though I knew I was overdressed. I wanted to make a good impression. Toward the end of the day, Craig told me that the dress code was very casual since all their clients and candidates were in the Bay Area and so never came into the office. The next day, I showed up in my favorite outfit: jeans and a black T-shirt. That became my daily uniform.

I spent the first week sitting at a desk next to Rick, learning everything I could about recruiting for software companies. He handed me a list of a bunch of software companies in the Bay Area and said that was their "hunting ground," the companies they focused on pulling people from. Then he handed me a list of his current clients and went over each one with me.

After that, we moved on to the résumés. He handed me a couple of examples. "These are good résumés."

I looked over one of them. "What makes them good?"

"These are software engineers, so I look first at where they went to school," he explained. "The second thing I look at is if they have worked at software companies. These people have graduated with engineering degrees from top schools and have worked at known software companies for the last five years—they'll be easy to place. You want to become very familiar with the list I gave you of all the top software companies in the Bay Area."

"Do you only place people who have worked at software companies before?" I asked.

"No. If someone is a salesperson or a marketer, it is a plus if they have worked at a software company, but it is not a must."

"So, what does a bad résumé look like?" I asked as I continued to look over the résumés.

Rick meticulously sifted through a stack of résumés and selected a few. "Here," he said, handing them over.

I scanned one and handed it back to him. "What's wrong with this one?"

"First off, they did not go to college," he said, pointing to the résumé's education section. "All of our clients prefer people who graduated from college. Second, they have never lasted more than a year in a company, and third, they have never worked at a software company. Companies are willing to pay us a fee because we give them people they can't find on a job board. They also want us to give them passive candidates."

"What do you mean by 'passive'?" I asked.

"I mean they want us to give them a currently employed candidate who is not actively 'looking' for a new job. Plus, they love it if we can get them someone who works for one of their competitors."

It was all starting to make sense to me.

Rick handed me an employee directory and a script. "Ready to make some phone calls?" he asked.

"Sure!"

I read the script a few times, then took a deep breath and dialed the number. It rang a few times, and the operator picked up.

"Hello, may I please be connected to Bob Anderson?" I asked.

I looked over at Rick as I waited to see if I would get connected.

Finally, I got connected to the number. Unfortunately, Bob did not answer his phone. I listened to Bob's voice message and waited nervously for the beep. When it sounded, I looked down at my script.

"Hello, Bob. Um . . . My name is Michael King. And . . . I'm with Littler Savage. Um . . . We recruit for both public software companies and startups in the Bay Area. If you have a minute, I would like to speak to you about some of the companies we work with and the roles I am working on!" I left him my phone number and wished him a great day, then hung up and took a deep breath.

"Not bad," Rick said with a curt nod. "But I want you to memorize the script and then put some of your personality into it, okay? You must make it sound like you are conversing with the person and not reading a script."

I wasn't sure I was ready to speak to an actual person just yet, so I was relieved to be sent to voice mail after voice mail over the next hour. Over that hour, I finally relaxed, and my messages started to sound more natural.

During my first week, I also sat next to Calvin and listened to him as he left voice messages and spoke to potential candidates. The days flew by, and I was off to the races.

I WAS A SPONGE in my first month on the job. I wanted to learn everything I could about the recruiting business. I would listen to the other recruiters when they left a voice message and when they had a candidate live on the phone. If they said something interesting, I wrote it down and tried to use it in my conversations. I also listened to Rick and Craig when they spoke to their clients, especially when negotiating an offer for one of their candidates.

I always kept my fingers crossed that someone would be interested in hearing about a new job. As the weeks went on, I got a couple of people to the interview stage for roles with Rick and Craig's clients, but no one got to the offer stage.

I know someone reading this today is probably thinking, *Wow, all I would have to do is go on LinkedIn, search for people who currently hold the role I am working on, and then send them an InMail to see if they're interested in a new job.*

Yes. Those were different times—the times of "dialing and emailing for dollars."

Even though I had not yet made a placement at Littler Savage, I was enjoying working there. The office was small, so there was lots of energy bouncing around in there, and it was cool when someone made a placement. It reminded me of playing baseball: when someone hit a home run, it was high fives all around.

I felt like things were starting to fall into place.

CHAPTER 51

IT WAS 7:47 P.M. on Wednesday, February 17, 1999, when Natalie Nicole King finally decided to make her appearance at Little Company of Mary Hospital in Torrance, California. She was nine days late—which, we would discover many years later, was a clue to her personality. Natalie liked to do things on her own timeline.

There in the operating room, Dr. Friedman presented Donnita and me with our eight-pound, nine-ounce, twenty-one-inch beautiful baby girl. We were both overjoyed.

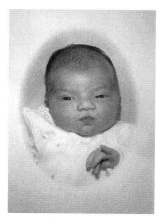

Natalie King

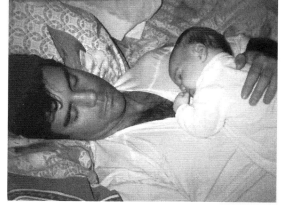

Me and Natalie

WHEN DONNITA WAS ready to return to work after Natalie's birth, we set up a system where she would drop Natalie off at my work and then drive to The Cheesecake Factory in Redondo Beach. When I left work, I would push Natalie down Santa Monica Boulevard to the parking garage in her stroller.

As the light turned green at the intersection one day, I began to push the stroller across the street. When we were halfway through the intersection, a voice called out on my right side, "Wow, what a beautiful baby!"

"Thank you."

I turned my head to see who thought I had a beautiful baby. It was Dustin Hoffman.

Celebrity encounters aside, it was very cool to be a dad. I was always excited to see Natalie when I came home from work. I loved holding and feeding her and even changing her diapers.

I was elated to welcome a little girl into my life—but I was simultaneously burdened by the weight of the responsibility it put on my shoulders. I felt it was my job to ensure that she and Donnita would have the life they deserved.

And even though I had not had a seizure in over a year, I was still very cautious when I held Natalie. *You never know*, I thought.

CHAPTER 52

A MONTH AFTER Natalie's birth, I finally made my first placement at Littler Savage: a software engineer at BroadVision. My commission on the placement was $6,000, just as Calvin had said it would be. Finally, I'd proven to myself that I could do this.

After that first placement in March, things started to pick up to a point where I was making a placement every month, and some months even two.

Since I'd grown up in the Bay Area, I decided to put together a list of questions that would help me connect with someone on the phone. When I found an appropriate time during my conversation with someone, I made sure to ask, "Did you grow up in the Bay Area?"

If they said no, my list of questions stopped. If they said yes, however, I followed up with "So did I. Where did you go to school?" If they grew up in the Bay Area (especially in San Francisco), they knew I meant what high school they attended, not what college—and the conversation usually took off from there.

One day, a guy I was speaking with told me he'd grown up in San Francisco and attended Riordan High School. "Really," I said. "Well, I can't talk to you then."

He was silent for a moment—and then he said, with an edge to his voice, "Really? Why? Did you go to SI?"

"Yes!" I said.

Riordan and St. Ignatius were fierce sports rivals. Our iciness was all in good fun, of course, and he and I ended up talking for about an hour about the people we knew in common. I told him that I'd played baseball at St. Ignatius, and he said he'd played football at Riordan. At the end of our conversation, he said he would send me his résumé and tell his coworkers about me.

I DIDN'T ATTEND St. Ignatius for all of high school—in fact, I didn't start there until my junior year. And if not for a chance encounter with a beautiful blonde named Patty Martin on a sunny September day at Thornton Beach in Daly City, I would never have transferred there.

Patty was beginning her junior year at Mercy High School in San Francisco, and I was starting my junior year at Westmoor High School in Daly City when we met. Mercy is a Catholic all-girls college-preparatory high school on 19th Avenue in San Francisco. Mercy and St. Ignatius were situated in the Sunset District of San Francisco, three miles from each other. I knew guys who went to St. Ignatius, and many dated girls from Mercy.

Patty was at the beach with some of her friends. After staring at her for an eternity, I finally found the guts to say hi. In the fall of 1976, I was not a "ladies' man." I had not even had a girlfriend yet, so I was extremely nervous around girls. But that day, when my buddies and I were ready to leave, I asked Patty for her phone number. To this day, I do not know how I got up the nerve to ask for her number—but I did.

For the next few weeks, she and I spoke on the phone. I liked her a lot and wanted to be able to call her my girlfriend. Sitting in my room after school one day, I started thinking about ways to make that happen.

"Dinner!" my mom called out from the kitchen, interrupting my thoughts.

I jumped off my bed and made my way to the dinner table. My dad and sister were already seated. My mom placed my plate in front of me. *Should I say something now?* I debated internally. *After dinner? Tomorrow?*

My mind was racing. I took a deep breath and then just went for it. "Dad, I want to transfer to SI!" I blurted out.

Our small kitchen became noticeably quiet.

My mom glanced at me with a mixture of surprise and curiosity, trying to gauge my sincerity.

My dad was shocked but happy at the same time. He had always wanted me to attend St. Ignatius, but I'd always insisted that I wasn't interested in attending an all-boys school. He gave me an appraising look. "What? Why do you want to transfer to SI?"

"I think I would get a better education at SI," I said. "Graduating from SI would also help me get into college; plus, having you as my pitching coach would be cool."

Karen rolled her eyes dramatically, sighed in exasperation, and said, "Oh, please."

But I'd convinced my dad. A big smile appeared on his face. "I'll call Art tomorrow."

Art Cecchin was the head of admissions and had worked for my dad at Flying Goose before joining St. Ignatius. With all my dad's connections at St. Ignatius, the transfer happened quickly.

Over the next two years, Patty and I went out a few times. Nothing romantic ever happened between us—but she did come with me to senior prom, and we had a wonderful time together that night.

Most of the time, the high school you graduate from does not have much bearing on your career—but in my case, graduating from St. Ignatius turned out to be a big plus for me. Since St. Ignatius is one of the top private schools in San Francisco, people often placed me in a particular category—automatically thought of me as smart—when I said I'd graduated from St. Ignatius. And now, all these years out of high school, it was helping me succeed at my new job.

CHAPTER 53

AT WORK, I CONTINUED TO try to find ways to bond with people over the phone. On the phone with a potential candidate one day, I asked if he'd grown up in the Bay Area. He said yes and told me he'd grown up in the Sunset District—the very neighborhood where my dad's sporting goods store was. I decided to mess with him a little.

"The Sunset," I said slowly. "Wasn't there a sporting goods store in the Sunset called "Flying . . ."

"Flying Goose!" he finished quickly.

"Yes! That was it," I replied. "Did you ever go there?"

"Yep—I loved that place. As a kid, I went there all the time. I got my Converse shoes, first baseball glove, and high school letterman jacket there. Great memories."

"Yeah, I probably waited on you a few times," I said.

He was quiet for a beat. Then it hit him. "Are you Tom King's son Mike?" he asked.

"Sure am," I said, laughing.

It turned out that my dad had coached him when he was in sixth grade. We talked about my dad and growing up in the Bay Area for the next hour.

With each cold call, I sensed a marked improvement in my ability to build meaningful connections with the people on the other end of the line in a relatively short time. I was learning.

IN JULY, RICK BOUGHT an updated employee directory for a company called Oracle in Redwood Shores, just south of San Francisco. He divided the directory into equal parts and handed the pieces to the recruiters.

Most of the calls I made to Oracle went directly to voice messages. About an hour into leaving messages, I decided to call one last person before going to the computer to send out some emails. I looked down at the next name on the list: Nancy Mills.

I dialed, asked for Nancy Mills, and waited for her recorded message. To my surprise, she answered the phone.

I recovered quickly and started my pitch—explaining what we did and what companies we worked with, and asking if she would be open to hearing about something new.

"Sure," she said. "May I have your email? I'll send you a message."

I rattled off my email address and was about to ask what she did at Oracle when she cut me short.

"Sorry, I have to jump into a meeting," she said. "But I'll send you my résumé first thing tomorrow morning, and if you have something for me, we can set up a call."

As I hung up the phone, I hoped with all my might that she was someone that I could place.

CHAPTER 54

I ARRIVED AT WORK early the next morning and immediately checked my email. There it was, the promised email from Nancy Mills.

I clicked on the attachment, and her résumé slowly appeared on my screen.

Nancy had almost twenty years of experience and had an impressive current title: Head of Professional Services – Consulting & Education. So far, most of the résumés I'd received were from people with somewhere between five and seven years of experience. This felt promising.

I printed out Nancy's résumé and handed it to Rick. His reaction to Nancy's résumé was similar to mine. He raised his eyebrows as he read through the CV, clearly impressed. "Good job, Michael!"

"Do you have anything for her?" I asked.

He mulled over options for a moment. "I think I'll reach out to the VP of HR at BroadVision," he said. BroadVision was Littler Savage's biggest client. They developed and sold software that allowed companies to identify online customers, retrieve data about purchases and online shopping habits, and personalize what customers saw on their websites. BroadVision had IPO'd in 1996, and now, three years later, the stock price had skyrocketed. They were one of the hottest tech companies in the Bay Area.

After Rick got off the phone with BroadVision, he approached my desk. "Here's the deal," he said. "I spoke to the VP of HR, and they have a retained search out for a VP of Professional Services role."

I had no clue what a "retained search" was. "What does that mean?"

He explained that a retained search was where a company paid a recruiting firm in advance to fill a specific role, unlike what we did—filling a role first, getting paid afterward. A company would pay a recruiting firm a chunk of money to start the search, usually one-third of the total fee. After the company had interviewed candidates and identified some top candidates, they paid the firm another third. The final third got paid out when the company hired a candidate for the role.

I want to do retained searches, I thought to myself. It sounded like a much better deal.

I noticed that Rick was starting to smile. "What's up?" I asked.

"Well, the VP of HR told me that the retained search firm had not given them any strong candidates in the last few weeks. She said that if we can find them a strong candidate, they'll look at them, and if they hire that candidate, we'll get paid."

Now *I* was smiling!

Rick handed me Nancy's résumé back. "See if she would be interested in a VP of professional services role at BroadVision."

I dashed to the nearest computer and wrote Nancy an email, asking if she was interested.

About an hour later, I received a response with only one word in the email: *Yes!*

I practically ran to Rick's desk. "She's interested," I said.

His face lit up. "Great! I'll get her right over there."

Just over a month later, I placed Nancy Mills as BroadVision's new VP of Professional Services. This was my first VP-level placement—the first VP-level placement by any recruiter at Littler Savage, in fact—and Rick and Craig decided to close the office early to commemorate my success. We celebrated at various bars along the Third Street Promenade.

My commission for the placement was $17,000—not bad for a few hours' work.

CHAPTER 55

YAMASHIRO, PERCHED IN THE Hollywood Hills, is a Japanese restaurant with spectacular panoramic views of LA from the Hollywood sign to the Pacific Ocean. Movie scenes have been shot there, and it's a stunning place: the exterior is modeled after a real castle in Japan, and it has both a beautiful Japanese garden that includes a giant Buddha statue and a striking garden courtyard with outdoor seating.

On this night, however, as Donnita and I celebrated my first VP placement, I wanted to sit at one of the window tables in the main dining room of my favorite sushi restaurant.

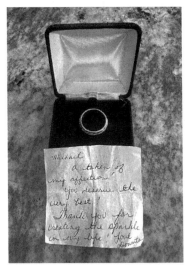

Over the next couple of hours, Donnita and I enjoyed lots of sushi—or should I say, I enjoyed lots of sushi. Donnita was always amazed at how much I could eat without gaining weight. We also enjoyed a few Sapporos and shots of sake.

As the server cleared our plates, I could tell Donnita was getting antsy. I was about to ask her what was going on when she reached into her purse, pulled out a wrapped box, and placed it in front of me.

"I love you," she said.

"What is it?" I asked.

She gestured toward the gift. "Open it."

The ring and note

I unwrapped the paper, opened the box, and found a smaller black box inside. A small yellow piece of paper, folded in half, was tucked under it. I unfolded the paper and read the note inside: *Michael, a token of my affection! You deserve the best! Thank you for creating the sparkle in my life! Love, Donnita*

In the box was a beautiful fourteen-karat gold wedding band with a silver twisted rope design.

"I thought that since you gave me a ring, you need one too," she said.

I placed the ring on my "wedding ring" finger, then gave her a big hug and kiss. "I love you!"

That night, I put the box and note in my nightstand drawer to keep them safe—and to this day, that's where they remain.

CHAPTER 56

IT WAS MID-OCTOBER when a letter arrived from the DMV. I was excited but also nervous to open it. Two months earlier, I'd had an appointment at UCLA with Dr. Mullin and asked him to fill out a Driver Medical Evaluation form for me for the DMV so I could get my license back. He'd said he would.

I had been taking the bus to Santa Monica for work for over a year, and Donnita had been driving me and Natalie everywhere. I needed to get my driver's license back.

I slowly opened the letter. "Yes!" I held up the letter for Donnita to see. "I can finally get my driver's license back!"

We hugged, and she let out a whoop. "Let's go to the DMV!"

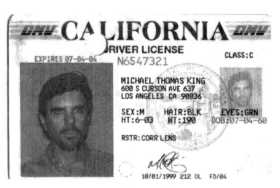

My new driver's license

WITH MY DRIVER'S license back in my wallet, I decided it was time to buy a car. My bartending buddy at Giggles, John, introduced me to the leasing and fleet manager at Sheridan Toyota in Santa Monica. A few days later, I drove there with Donnita and drove off the lot an hour later with a gold 1998 Toyota Camry with ten thousand miles on it.

I was a bit nervous the first time I got back behind the wheel, but after driving a few times, the anxiety went away.

A few weeks after we picked up my new car, Donnita wanted to go to a party at her friend's house in Redondo Beach. Since she had been stuck driving me around since my accident, I insisted on driving her there.

We had a fun time at the party; I knew a few of her friends, and they were excited to hear that I was doing well after my surgeries. Since I was driving, I made sure that I only had one beer.

When it was time to head back home, I decided to take Aviation Boulevard̩K. As we made our way down Aviation, Donnita said, "You can make a right on Manhattan Beach and catch the 405 if you want."

"I know." I continued down Aviation, past Manhattan Beach Boulevard.

"You just passed Manhattan Beach," Donnita said.

"I know. I need to see something."

Two blocks later, we approached Rosecrans, where I'd crashed my car.

I slowed down as we passed Rosecrans and glanced over the trees to the right where I'd crashed. A wave of emotions welled up within me. This was the first time I had returned to the place where I'd totaled my car and could have lost my life. I could still feel Donnita's eyes on me.

"Are you okay?" she asked.

"I'm good. I just had to do this." I reached over, held her hand, and then kissed it.

I turned right on El Segundo Boulevard, got on the 405, and headed home.

CHAPTER 57

IT WAS THE last few weeks of 1999. My goal for my first full year at Littler Savage had been to make $100K. I came up a bit short—I made $60,750—but this was still significant for me, since I had only been averaging $18,000 yearly since being diagnosed with epilepsy.

I felt confident that I could make over $100K as a recruiter, so I started to look over the homes for sale in the real estate section whenever I read the Sunday *LA Times*. I knew we were a long way away from being able to buy a house, but if I could consistently make over $100K a year, our dream might come true.

I went through 1999 seizure-free. In December, I asked Dr. Mullin if we could lower my medication. "The Tegretol makes me so tired and lethargic," I complained. "I just want to have more energy."

"I understand, Michael, but I'm uncomfortable lowering my dosage at this time," he told me. "For now, I want to keep you at seventeen hundred milligrams."

I finally received the bill from UCLA for my stay in the hospital from December 16, 1997, to January 4, 1998 (two invasive EEGs and the surgery). It came to $132,483. All told, my two visits to UCLA came to a total of $156,180.

Even though the medical and credit card bills were piling up, I knew things would work out for our little family. I was looking forward to having a big 2000.

CHAPTER 58

JANUARY 30, 2000. The countertop of our small apartment was lined with chicken wings, nachos, sliders, guacamole, and an assortment of chips. Two coolers were on the floor next to the countertop, filled with beers and sodas. Super Bowl XXXIV, to be played between the St. Louis Rams and the Tennessee Titans, was about to start, and our apartment was crowded with a bunch of our friends.

The game was exhilarating, especially the ending, when Titans receiver Kevin Dyson stretched for the goal line with no time remaining, and Rams linebacker Mike Jones wrapped his arms around Dyson and brought him down one yard short of the goal line.

The ending was exciting, but the most exciting part of the Super Bowl for me was all the tech company commercials. During the previous Super Bowl, a total of only two tech company commercials had aired. During this one I counted *seventeen*, and each company had spent more than $2 million on advertising, earning Super Bowl XXXIV the nickname the "Dot-com Super Bowl."

The two most memorable commercials for me were E*TRADE (a dancing monkey and two men clapped to music as the caption read, "Well, we just wasted $2 million. What are you doing with your money?") and Budweiser (Rex the dog recalls his worst day).

The economy was doing great, and tech companies were leading the charge. Priceline, which had IPO'd in March of 1999, was trading at around $162 a share at the start of the year. The price had been $16 a share before the IPO. Meanwhile, CommerceOne stock was trading at $218 a share, with a market value of $20 billion, and in February BroadVision's stock was trading at $240 a share (and that was after a three-for-one stock split in October of 1999—they would have another three-for-one stock split in March of 2000). In March 2000, InfoSpace stock was at $1,305 per share. On March 10, 2000, the NASDAQ Composite Stock Market Index peaked at 5,048.62.

Tech was hot, and I felt so lucky to be recruiting in this industry.

It was an exciting time to recruit for tech companies in the Bay Area. It was like shooting fish in a barrel. I could not find candidates fast enough for our clients. Rick and Craig decided to subscribe to Dice so we could find candidates more quickly than calling employee directories all day would allow.

There were too many tech jobs and not enough qualified candidates looking for jobs, so companies were competing to hire top talent. Some companies decided to stretch the truth on how well they were doing to impress candidates.

Another company decided to take things a step further.

MY PHONE RANG at work one day. I picked it up immediately. "Hello?"

It was a candidate of mine that I had scheduled a second-round interview at a fast-growing startup for. "They locked me in!" he said.

"What?" I asked, astonished.

"They locked me into the conference room so I couldn't leave," he said, and then explained further.

During his interview, one of the company executives had asked him if he was interviewing with other companies, and he'd told him the truth: he was talking to two other companies, and they were moving quickly. The executive had asked him if he could stay longer and meet two more people. He'd said yes. After he'd met with them, the hiring manager had returned, given him a written offer to sign, and left the conference room—locking the door behind him.

The hiring manager finally unlocked the door and let my candidate out of the conference room. After that experience, understandably, he did not accept their offer. Luckily, I placed him at another company.

AS THE RÉSUMÉ from a candidate I had recently spoken to began to download, I thought, *Wow! I should be able to place her quickly!* With a BS degree from Stanford and an MBA from Stanford, she had the perfect pedigree. I started to count my money before I even decided where we should have her interview.

It was not long before I had her set up for a round of interviews with

Informatica, one of Rick's clients. Informatica loved her, and she was interested in the role and the company. Cha-ching!

A day before her final interview, however, she called to let me know that she was interviewing with another company and they wanted to make her an offer. I asked her to tell me more about the company. She said it was a small startup. She was torn. She liked the opportunity at Informatica, but the startup was founded by two ex-Stanford graduates, plus there were other employees at the company who'd also gone to Stanford. She described the role she was being offered there. It was not as senior a role as the one at Informatica, but she felt there was lots of potential.

"What's the name of the company?" I asked.

"Google," she said.

She ended up going to Google. I am sure she is retired on an island somewhere now.

CHAPTER 59

SINCE 2000 STARTED on fire, Rick and Craig decided to add another recruiter, Andrew, to our team. Less than a month after Andrew started, he made his first placement. It was late on a Friday afternoon when a client called Craig to inform him that Andrew's candidate had sent her signed offer letter back. When Craig got off the phone, he gave Andrew the good news.

Andrew was so excited. I gave him a big high five and handed him a dry-erase pen to put his first placement on the whiteboard that showed all our placements for the quarter.

"We need to go celebrate!" Craig said. "We're closing early today."

We headed to the Third Street Promenade and celebrated into the night.

EVERYONE WAS IN great spirits when we returned to the office on Monday. Until Andrew checked his email.

"FUCK!" he yelled, staring at the computer screen.

Everyone's attention turned to him.

He exhaled loudly. "She fucking changed her mind and is going to take another offer."

Craig moved to the computer to read the email. The candidate had written that one of the references she'd given to our client—an ex-boss from a previous company who was now working at a hot startup—had called her over the weekend. He had not been aware that she was looking to make a move until he got the reference call, and now that he was, he wanted her. He'd offered her more money and a bigger title if she joined his company. Of course, she'd said yes.

Andrew walked over to the board and erased his deal. He never recovered from that day. Six months later, he left the company and the recruiting business for good.

When people ask me what the most challenging part of being a recruiter is, I tell them it's not finding candidates or opening a new client—it's dealing with the emotional highs and lows. After witnessing what happened to Andrew, I realized that in order to succeed in business and in life, you must know how to control your emotions. You can never get too high or too low.

I was off to a great start in 2000. In the first three months, I'd made at least two placements a month; one month, I'd even made three. I was well on my way to making over $100K for the year.

Since things were going so well, I decided to finally quit my bartending job at Giggles.

CHAPTER 60

UPON RETURNING TO the office from a late lunch on Friday, April 14, 2000, my attention was immediately drawn to Rick and Craig, who were engaged in a serious conversation at the back of the office. While Rick spoke, Craig repeatedly shook his head, and I found myself unable to resist stealing repeated glances in their direction as I settled back at my desk.

"What's going on?" I asked Calvin.

"Rick said that the stock market is crashing today, and many tech companies are leading it," he said grimly.

This was news to me; I started searching online for news and quickly found plenty of it.

The Nasdaq had shed 355.61 points, or over 9 percent, dropping down to 3,321.17. The Index had lost over 1,000 points the week of April 14 and was off more than 34 percent from the record high on March 10. Wall Street had seen a 20 percent decline in the market as the beginning of a bear market. They were calling it "Black Friday."

Was this just a bad week and the market would bounce back?

We all hoped so.

EVEN THOUGH THE market was crashing, some of our clients were still hiring. In August 2000, I placed my second VP at BroadVision, a VP of WW Corporate Marketing.

Rick and Craig tried to stay optimistic that things would turn around.

By November 2000, however, things were even worse. News broke that Pets.com was shutting down only nine months after its IPO. The Bloomberg US Internet Index calculated that 280 stocks had fallen to $1.2 trillion from $2.9 trillion at their peak, a loss of $1.7 trillion.

By the end of the year, Amazon stock had lost more than 75 percent of its value. InfoSpace stock slid steadily, reaching just $13.69 on December 10, a 95 percent drop. Priceline stock declined 99 percent to under $6. CommerceOne was now trading at $35 a share.

I ended the year at $81,500. If things had not slowed down at the end of the year, I would have made my target—but as things were, that $100K mark still remained elusive.

I wanted to stay positive that things would bounce back, but it was hard to stay positive when I noticed that more and more of our clients were no longer hiring.

Health-wise, it was a great year: I remained seizure-free and Natalie was thriving, getting bigger every day. I was disappointed that Dr. Mullin still wanted me to stay on the same dosage, but grateful that I was otherwise doing well.

Eagerly awaiting the arrival of 2001, I could never have fathomed the extraordinary twists and formidable challenges that would unfold for our family in the coming year.

CHAPTER 61

As DONNITA AND I watched Super Bowl XXXV between the New York Giants and the Baltimore Ravens in our apartment on January 28, 2001, it quickly became evident that tech companies' advertising craziness during the Super Bowl had slowed down. Only three tech companies—E*TRADE, HotJobs, and Monster—aired commercials, and unsurprisingly (since tech companies were having massive layoffs), two of the three were job-hunting companies.

E*TRADE decided to take a jab at the darling of the 2000 Super Bowl, Pets.com, as the E*TRADE chimp rode into a ghost town of dot.com advertisers from the previous year holding the sock puppet character from Pets.com with a tear rolling down its cheek.

As I watched the Ravens crush the Giants 34–7, I could not stop thinking about how quickly things had changed for me and our family. I really thought I had found my calling as a recruiter. I knew I had to stay optimistic that things would improve, but it was hard. It seemed like every day a new client was letting Rick and Craig know that roles were on hold or they were no longer using outside recruiters. They kept scrambling to find new clients who would work with us and were trying to keep our current clients by lowering our fee structure, but it felt like a losing battle.

DURING THE FIRST six months of 2001, I only made two placements, and my commission was lower than usual since Rick and Craig had lowered our fees.

Donnita and I had a vacation coming up that we had been planning for over a year. Even though the money was tight and it was not the best time for either of us to take a break from work, we decided to go ahead with the trip. We needed the break.

CHAPTER 62

IN AUGUST, WE PACKED Donnita's Ford Explorer and headed to Lake Tahoe for a family vacation and reunion with my side of the family. My parents, my sister, and her kids, Nick, Matt, and Leya, would all be there, as would my cousins Eric and John and my uncle Tom and aunt Penny, whom I hadn't seen for a few years. I looked forward to playing golf with my cousins and uncle at Edgewood Golf Course and the Incline Village Championship Golf Course.

As you can imagine, the star of the trip was none other than Natalie. She was two and a half years old now, and everyone wanted to hold and play with her.

The trip was going great until I received a call from Rick, letting me know that we'd be having an all-hands meeting on Monday morning when I returned from Tahoe. As I hung up the phone, my mind raced about what would be discussed at the meeting. Were they letting go of one or two of us recruiters? Were things turning around? Were they going to try to recruit in a different industry?

For the remainder of our time in Tahoe, I couldn't stop thinking about that meeting.

AS SOON AS I walked into the office on Monday morning, I knew the meeting was not going to end on a positive note. The looks on the faces of the other recruiters let me know that Rick and Craig had already shared the news with them.

I sat down in a chair next to Calvin, and the room fell silent.

Rick and Craig stood before us. Rick spoke first. He did not sugarcoat anything.

"We've decided to shut down the office," he said bluntly. "All of our clients have made it clear that they won't be using outside recruiters for the remainder of the year—even BroadVision won't be doing any hiring for quite a while."

This wasn't a surprise; BroadVision's stock was in a freefall. By the end of that year, BroadVision stock would lose 75 percent and end up at $1.25 per share.

It was now Craig's time to speak. "We're not giving up on this," he said. "Rick and I will continue to try to open new clients, and any time we find roles for you to work on, we'll let you know. We encourage you to work from home and try to find companies that are hiring. And stay connected with candidates you have placed too, in case they hear about companies that are hiring."

We finally packed up our stuff, exchanged hugs, and said our good-byes. Only two and a half years earlier, I'd been excited to become a tech recruiter. Now what?

AUGUST WAS A very tough month. I was at a crossroads. Should I continue down this same path, or should I try something new?

Whatever I was going to do, I had to figure it out quickly. We needed *two* incomes to pay our bills.

CHAPTER 63

DONNITA AND I had been talking about whether or not we should bring Natalie up in LA since the day she was born. Since Donnita hadn't had the best experience growing up in LA, she was not thrilled about bringing up our daughter there. I, meanwhile, had seen a lot in my fifteen years in the city—everything from girls being taken advantage of as they tried to break into the entertainment industry to underaged girls being allowed into nightclubs.

Before things had started to slow down in my job, and it looked like I could continually make $100K a year, the discussion about leaving LA had trickled to a stop. But now that things had changed and I couldn't find any companies looking to hire a tech recruiter in LA, the discussion started up again.

One day, after I spent over an hour on Dice looking for tech-recruiting roles in LA, I decided to see if there were any in the San Francisco Bay Area, since the Bay Area was the "tech hub" of the US. I quickly found multiple listings—both recruiting agencies looking to hire tech recruiters and tech companies looking to hire recruiters.

But if we were going to move to the Bay Area or anywhere else, Donnita would also need to find a job. I knew The Cheesecake Factory had opened a restaurant on top of the Macy's building in Union Square in San Francisco in 2000; maybe she could transfer there?

Going back home sounded very appealing, but where would we live? I knew we could not afford a place in San Francisco, so that was out of the question. We could afford a place in Concord, where my parents lived, but how would Donnita get to work? The idea of her having to drive over an hour into San Francisco or take BART (train system) to work didn't sound too appealing.

During dinner one night, Donnita threw out another option: "What about moving to Seattle? There's a Cheesecake Factory there."

Donnita's parents lived only two and a half hours from Seattle in Wenatchee; her younger sister, Becky, lived on Bainbridge Island, a thirty-five-minute ferry ride from Seattle; and her aunt Joanne lived in Seattle proper. But I'd left the fog of San Francisco for the warm weather of LA for a reason; I wasn't sure that Seattle was the place for me.

"Seattle? Doesn't it rain all the time there?" I asked.

"No!" Donnita insisted. "And it would be great if Natalie could be around my family; plus, it's more affordable than the Bay Area." I could see the wheels spinning as she thought it all through. "I can call David Overton tomorrow and see if I can transfer to the Seattle restaurant. He always told me to let him know if I ever needed anything."

David was the owner of The Cheesecake Factory. Donnita had worked for the company since 1992, when she was hired at the Newport Beach location—their fourth location to open. During the early days, David had sometimes made surprise visits to the Newport location, and he had always complimented Donnita on her work ethic and considered her a valued employee. If ever there was a time to take him up on his offer, this seemed like it.

THE NEXT DAY, Donnita called David, who immediately agreed to let her transfer to the Seattle restaurant and then move over to the newest restaurant when it opened in Bellevue, Washington, in January.

I knew nothing about the greater Seattle area. "Where's Bellevue?"

"David said it was ten miles east of Seattle," she said with a little shrug. "It must be a nice area if he wants to open a restaurant there. I also told him that I was looking to get out of bartending and was interested in the bookkeeper job in Bellevue, and he said it was mine if I wanted it. I told him I wanted it."

Donnita was excited to get back to a nine-to-five job. She had kept the books for her ex-husband's company for many years and enjoyed it. She smirked at me. "Looks like *I* have a job. Now *you* need to find one!"

I had never been afraid to pick up and move. While Seattle was not a place I'd ever really wanted to live, I was open to trying it out if I could find a job.

"I'll start looking," I promised.

CHAPTER 64

On September 1, 2001, I logged on to my computer in the bedroom and went to Dice to see if any companies were looking for a technical recruiter in the Seattle area. Not surprisingly, there were not as many companies looking for tech recruiters there as there were in the Bay Area—but there were a couple. I immediately applied online.

Over the next week, more openings in the Seattle area popped up. I applied for each one and never got a response. That surprised me at first, but after thinking about it more, it made sense: I had only been recruiting for just over two years, and before that, I'd been a bartender. I was sure the companies must be responding to people with more recruiting experience than me.

One day, I shared my frustrations with Donnita. I was not surprised by her response.

"Do you really still want to be a recruiter?" she nudged me. "Why don't you try something different? You are good at sales. Maybe a sales job somewhere."

I felt like I was back in 1998 again, when Donnita was pregnant and I first set out to find a day job.

I decided to apply for sales jobs in the Seattle area in every industry imaginable.

Still no responses.

One night, I couldn't sleep, so I decided to log on to Dice. I still felt attached to being a recruiter; I really enjoyed the work. *Maybe some new tech-recruiting jobs have opened up in Seattle since I last looked*, I thought hopefully.

After scrolling through some jobs, I came across a job posting from a company called Triad Group. They were looking for a technical recruiter, and the office was in Bellevue.

I looked over at Donnita in bed. She was sleeping, but seemingly not very soundly. I walked over and knelt in front of her.

"Hey," I softly said.

Donnita slowly opened her eyes. "What?"

"Was Bellevue the city where the new Cheesecake was opening up?" I asked.

"Yes . . . Why?"

"Never mind. I will tell you later. Go back to sleep."

I strode back to my desk and read the job description. Then I pulled up Triad Group's website. While looking it over, I noticed they had been in business since 1986. If they had been around for that long and were still open and hiring, I figured, it must be a stable company. I decided to apply. I crossed my fingers as I submitted the application form.

TWO DAYS LATER, the phone rang. It was someone from Triad Group. They said they'd received my résumé, and the owner, Jim Mercer, wanted to set up a call to discuss the technical recruiting role with me. I spoke to the person briefly, then hung up and gave Donnita the excellent news.

Jim and I spoke the next day. During our call, he mentioned that all of Triad Group's clients were located in the Seattle area, and said he liked the fact that I had recruited for tech companies in Silicon Valley. After speaking for forty-five minutes, he invited me to come to the Bellevue office and meet with him. We agreed on a 10:00 a.m. meeting on Wednesday, September 26.

After hanging up the phone, I eagerly shared the fantastic news with Donnita, who could not contain her excitement about relocating to Seattle and being nearer to her family. The timing could not have been more ideal, especially considering that Rick and Craig had decided to close down Littler Savage at the beginning of September.

AT 6:00 A.M. on September 11, the phone rang. I had slept in Natalie's bedroom that night so Donnita and Natalie could have a mother-daughter sleepover in our bedroom. I got up and made my way to the phone in the kitchen.

The second I picked up, Donnita's sister Becky's frantic voice shouted through the receiver, "Did you guys see what happened? I heard they are targeting Los Angeles next."

Since I was still half asleep, I was not 100 percent sure what she was saying. "What?" I asked groggily.

"Turn on the news!" she said.

I made my way over to the TV and turned it on. Immediately, the image of a high-rise filled with smoke filled the screen; then, as I watched in horror, a plane crashed into the high-rise next to the first smoke-filled skyscraper.

"What the fuck is going on?" I asked.

"That's the second plane to crash into the World Trade Center," Becky said.

"I have to get Donnita!" I hung up and ran to wake her up.

For the next five days we mostly sat in front of the TV, trying to comprehend what we were seeing.

CHAPTER 65

ON TUESDAY, SEPTEMBER 25, I landed in Seattle. The first thing I noticed was the bright blue sky. The last time I'd seen a sky so blue was in Lake Tahoe. The second thing I noticed was the temperature outside—it was eighty-eight degrees.

I got my rental car and was about to get on the freeway when I noticed a large snow-capped mountain on the horizon. It looked so close that I thought about checking it out—but when I looked on a map, I realized it was Mount Rainier, which was a full seventy-one miles from the Seattle airport. *Maybe later*, I thought, chuckling to myself, and decided to check into my hotel.

WHEN I ARRIVED at the Triad Group office the following morning, I immediately noticed that it was about three times the size of the Littler Savage office. After I introduced myself to the office manager at the front desk, she walked me back to Jim's office.

As we strolled through the office, I couldn't help but notice that each person had their own office—a stark contrast to the setup at Littler Savage, where we all sat close together in a small shared room.

Jim and I sat in his office and talked for a good hour. I told him about the companies I'd recruited for in the Bay Area and the distinct roles I'd placed at those companies. He asked me about my recruiting style and how I sourced candidates. I gave him the full rundown on how things had worked at Littler Savage.

As our conversation ended, he asked me to send him three references. "Assuming everything goes well with your references," he added, "when would you be able to start?"

"The beginning of November," I said.

"That should be perfect," he said.

We shook hands, and he walked me out to the front door.

As soon as I got to my car, I called Donnita and told her that the meeting had gone well; I felt confident he would offer me the job. She was excited for me and us.

DONNITA HAD SUGGESTED that I stay a few extra days in Seattle to visit with her family and do some apartment hunting, and that's exactly what I did. After one day on Bainbridge Island with Becky's family, I took the ferry back to Seattle and drove around the downtown area. I immediately felt that Seattle was similar to San Francisco: a fisherman's wharf filled with seafood restaurants, tourist traps, and one-way streets.

I spent my final two days driving around the Seattle area, looking at apartments with Donnita's parents. She'd insisted that I bring my video camera along so she could get an idea of what the places I'd toured looked like, so everywhere we went I pulled out the camera and took some video.

During my interview with Jim, he'd mentioned that I should look at apartments in Kirkland—an area located seven miles from Bellevue that had a downtown waterfront area with a marina, restaurants, and shops. It was quaint and picturesque and reminded me a lot of Sausalito, California.

After looking at apartments around Bellevue and Kirkland, we headed east on the I-90 freeway to Issaquah, a growing area twelve miles from Bellevue that had a good-size lake, Lake Sammamish.

By the time I boarded the plane and returned to LA, I was feeling great about my trip. I'd had a great interview; I'd taken a ferry ride, gotten lost in downtown Seattle, checked out apartments in Bellevue, Kirkland, and Issaquah, and enjoyed four sunny days in the high eighties. As the plane took off, I thought, *Why does everyone say it always rains in Seattle?*

CHAPTER 66

ONCE BACK HOME, I showed Donnita the video footage of the apartments. She was excited about some of them, especially the one in Kirkland—The Preserve at Forbes Creek. She liked that there were three swimming pools and two hot tubs and that the top-floor units had a view of the Olympic Mountains. She also liked the fact that it was only nine miles from Bellevue.

She was getting really excited about the possibility of moving to Seattle. I was cautiously optimistic; I hoped that I would hear from Jim soon.

JUST A FEW days after I got back from Seattle, Jim called and offered me a job as a recruiter at Triad Group. Of course, I said yes! We agreed on compensation and a start date of Monday, November 19. Donnita had her transfer to the Seattle Cheesecake Factory confirmed and set to start on the same day I would begin my new job. I was excited about starting a new job and discovering a new city.

October was filled with planning for our move. We decided to go with the apartment in Kirkland—and since the economy was still in a recession, they offered us one month of free rent. We got a three-bedroom, two-bath apartment on the top floor of the building, facing the Olympic Mountains, for $1,300 a month. We found a company to pack and transport our stuff to Kirkland.

Donnita and I decided she and Natalie would take the train to Seattle. I would drive my car, and her dad, Gerry, would follow me in her car from LA to Sacramento, Sacramento to Oregon, and then Oregon to our new apartment in Kirkland. Once Donnita and Natalie arrived in Seattle, Becky would take them back to her place on Bainbridge Island, where they would stay until Gerry and I arrived in Kirkland on November 5, the same day the movers were scheduled to arrive.

It was all coming together.

- - -

I HAD ONE last thing to do before I could leave for Seattle.

A week before we left, I met with Dr. Mullin to let him know I was moving to Seattle. He gave me the names of two neurologists in Seattle, just in case I started to have seizures again, and also gave me some good news: "Since you've been seizure-free since the operation, I want to lower your daily dosage to sixteen hundred milligrams," he told me. "So just twice a day now—two four-hundred-milligram pills in the morning and two in the evening. Make sure to always take the correct daily dosage!"

"I will," I assured him. I was thrilled to reduce my dosage by any amount.

"Have you experienced any other short-term or long-term memory loss since we last spoke?"

"Not that I'm aware of," I said. (Donnita later reminded me that I had forgotten some important dates and names of people and places, but at the time I genuinely didn't remember that.)

Before we parted ways, Dr. Mullin dropped a bombshell: "You know, this was the first MST to be performed at UCLA," he told me. "We're so thrilled you're doing so well."

Hearing this for the first time, my jaw almost hit the floor. But I wasn't angry; after all, knowing that fact before my surgery wouldn't have changed my mind about wanting the procedure done. I'd been ready to try anything to cure my epilepsy.

I recently learned that MST surgery is rarely done even today. As Donnita likes to say, "You are a miracle, Michael!"

Dr. Mullin wished me good luck and told me to call him if I ever needed to talk. I hugged him and thanked him for everything he had done for me.

Seattle, here we come!

CHAPTER 67

ON SATURDAY, NOVEMBER 6, I left LA in my overstuffed Toyota Camry, Gerry following behind in Donnita's Ford Explorer. As I ascended the Grapevine on the 405, I realized that my dream of becoming an actor or writer in Hollywood had officially reached its conclusion.

As a kid, I never thought about becoming an actor or model. I always wanted to be a professional baseball player. But during the fall term of my senior year at St. Mary's College, my life took an unexpected turn.

I needed to take a religious studies class to graduate. I'd heard from numerous people that Brother Matthew Benney's class was the class to take, if you could get in, so I tried to register for the class . . . but it was full. My only option was to simply show up for the class the first day and see if there was room for any additional students.

That first morning, Brother Matthew entered the room and read off the names of the students who had registered for his class. He then looked at everyone against the back wall and asked us to say something about ourselves and why we needed to add his class. After everyone gave their best "sob story," I went for a different approach: I calmly explained that I was from Daly City and played baseball, and this was the only religious studies course that fit into my class schedule.

The next day, my name was on the list of people he was accepting into his class.

At the end of my first day in Brother Matthew's class, just as I started to walk out of the classroom, he called out, "Michael! Can you stick around for a few minutes?"

"Sure, Brother Matthew." I sat down at one of the desks and waited.

"Do you know anything about St. Mary's drama department?" he asked me.

"Not really," I said, unsure where the conversation was headed.

"Well, in addition to religious studies, I teach drama and direct plays here at the school," he said. "Have you ever thought about getting into acting?"

He caught me off guard with that question. "No," I said honestly. "Not really."

"Well, would you be open to attending one of my evening classes and seeing if it might interest you?"

My interest was piqued. "Sure! Why not?"

After that day, Brother Matthew took me under his wing. He introduced me to great plays, worked with me on monologues, and engaged me in long conversations about what it took to be an actor. On one occasion, Brother Matthew asked me if I wouldn't mind picking up someone from the airport. It was an actor friend from LA who was going to speak to our class. Of course, I said yes. Later that day, Harry Hamlin stood on the stage and talked to our class about being an actor. When I graduated, Brother Matthew helped me get my first agent in San Francisco. But most importantly, he made me fall in love with acting.

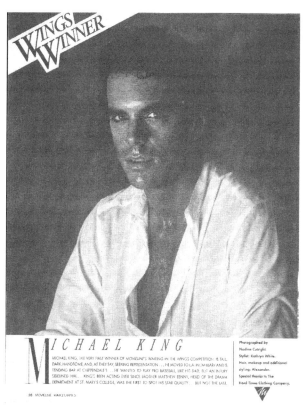

Waiting in the Wings

BE THERE WHEN I RETURN

--- --- ---

WHEN I MOVED to LA in January 1986, things started to happen for me almost immediately. In March, I appeared in *Movieline* magazine as the first winner of a contest they called "Waiting in the Wings." That exposure helped me get a theatrical and a commercial agent.

A year later, after moving into my first apartment on Larrabee just below Sunset in West Hollywood, I came home from a night of bartending at Chippendales and was surprised to see that my answering machine was full of messages. I rewound the small cassette tape and hit Play—and listened as message after message from random guys asking for a female date for the night filled the air. After answering a call the next day from a guy also looking for a date, I looked at the Yellow Pages and discovered that the number the phone company had given me had formerly belonged to the Beverly Hills Escort Service. After changing my number, I told a guy I got to know in my acting class about what had happened. He had the same thought I was having: *We need to write a screenplay about this!*

We had a completed screenplay a few months later, and I had the perfect title for it: *It Happened for a Reason*. Not long after that, I started chatting with a woman who came in and sat at the bar for lunch when I was working at the Hard Rock, and found out that she was a script reader for Creative Artists Agency (CAA).

I figured I had nothing to lose, so I went for it—"Have I got a script for you!"

As I started telling her the story, she giggled and then laughed. After hearing my pitch, she handed me her card. "Bring the script by, and I'll have someone read it," she said.

The next day, I dropped off the script at CAA.

OVER THE NEXT few months, I would go from the highest of highs to the lowest of lows.

The initial reader's report Suzanne showed me was incredibly positive: *The plot is complex but is also well thought out and developed. The twists are great. Overall, the script is worth considering.*

Next, I was told that two actors CAA represented, James Spader and

C. Thomas Howell, and a director they represented, Daniel Petrie Jr., were interested in the script.

But then I got the feedback that when the script was sent to producers, they kept hearing that my story was too similar to *Risky Business* and *Night Shift*.

Ultimately, nothing materialized with CAA, and although I kept showing people my script, nothing happened with it. I wrote two more scripts after that, but there was no interest in making either one into a movie.

Creative Artist's Agency, Inc.

READER'S REPORT

Title: IT HAPPENED FOR A REASON

Submitted to: SA
From: SUZANNE UNREIN

Author: ARTHUR G. POUNSFORD & MICHAEL KING

Purpose of
Submission: GENERAL

Publisher:

Reader: TED MILLER

Type: 122 pp. Screenplay

Date: 4/6/88

Time & Location: PRESENT: LOS ANGELES

Motion Picture Meeting

Fri. Material Meeting

Creative Meeting

Fri. Book Meeting   Other

THEME

CHRIS EDWARDS, mid-twenties and fed up with living in a small town, decides to move to Los Angeles to join his best friend from high school, JEFF NOBLE, on the road to success.

Readers Report – Cover Page

COMMENTS:

"It Happened for a Reason" is a terrifically unpredictable screenplay. It successfully combines elements of of drama, mystery and humor to make a wonderful script.
The characters, all very diverse, are interesting and well developed. The characters of Jeff and Chris, for example, are entertaining and offer terrific roles for males in their mid-twenties. Jeff is a high energy entrepreneur who is ultimately the driving force behind the duo's adventures while Chris, who is a bit naive at first, develops into the adventuresome, but more cautious, of the duo.

The plot is complex, but is also well thought out and developed. The twists are great.

Overall, the script is worth considering.

Readers Report - Comments

I went on numerous auditions for movies, TV shows, and soap operas, but despite my best efforts, I never managed to book anything. Every time I went on an audition, the room was filled with guys that looked like me. The competition was fierce. I just wanted a chance. I was able to book print jobs for companies like Mercedes Benz and Yamaha, and I played the boyfriend of country singer Mila Mason in the music video for her debut single, "That's Enough of That."

But I never really got my big break, and eventually I shifted my focus to other things.

As I wound my way up through the Grapevine, I made my peace with the fact that my Hollywood dreams hadn't panned out.

I guess it wasn't meant to be.

CHAPTER 68

ON MONDAY, NOVEMBER 5, I pulled into our new apartment complex in Kirkland, Washington, with Gerry close behind. The movers were already busy unloading our stuff. As I pulled into a parking spot and parked my car, I turned my windshield wipers from "high" to "off." It was pouring rain.

I could not help but feel like Mother Nature had played a sly trick on me. The weather had been amazing when I was in Seattle only two months earlier. But from the time we moved there through the next six months, it seemed like it rained every day. If it had been like that when I'd interviewed, I'm not sure I would have wanted to move there. I was here now, though, so I had to make the best of it.

Gerry and I stepped into the apartment and were greeted by the sight of Donnita diligently unpacking boxes. It was great to see my girls.

Within hours, everything was moved into our apartment.

DONNITA'S MOM ARRIVED the following day. She and Gerry stayed with us for two days, helping unpack, before they headed back to Wenatchee. As they were leaving, Gerry left us with these important words: "You need to get Washington license plates immediately. You do not want to be driving around with California license plates."

But we had an extensive list of things we needed to get done before starting our jobs, so we put "get new license plates" on the back burner. We figured we had time.

TWO WEEKS AFTER starting our new jobs, we decided to visit Donnita's parents in Wenatchee. Donnita wanted to drive, so we took her Ford Explorer.

About forty-five minutes into our drive on I-90 East, Donnita noticed a dirty sedan following her.

She looked into the rearview mirror. "There's a car behind me with disco lights flashing on their dashboard."

I looked in the side mirror and saw the red and blue flashing lights on the car's dashboard. "Is that a cop car?"

She squinted into the mirror. "I don't know."

"I think you're getting pulled over," I said.

As Donnita pulled over and put the car in park, I looked in my side mirror. The car door opened, and a state trooper stepped out. He placed his "Smokey the Bear" hat on his head as he made his way to our car. As he walked up to Donnita's side of the car, I thought, *I should have listened to Gerry and gotten Washington license plates.*

The officer asked for the registration and Donnita's license. She told him we had just moved to Washington, hoping that might earn us a little grace. No such luck; he returned a minute later with a speeding ticket.

After that encounter with a Washington state trooper, I always slowed down when I saw a dirty sedan behind me, afraid it might be a state trooper in an unmarked car.

CHAPTER 69

ON MONDAY, NOVEMBER 19, Donnita drove to the Seattle Cheesecake Factory on the corner of 7th Avenue and Pike Street, where she began training for a new role as a "store accounting technician," and I headed to Triad Group for my first day of work.

That first day was eye-opening. I wore dress pants and a dress shirt to work—much different from the attire I was used to at Littler Savage. I missed wearing my jeans-and-T-shirt uniform already.

Jim showed me to my new office when I arrived, and it was huge; all four recruiters at Littler Savage could have fit into the space. I felt strange being all alone in there. With everyone in their own offices, the entire floor was quiet.

As a bartender and as a recruiter, I had always been around people—and I loved it. I fed off the energy of others. Now, alone in a private office, I would have to find a way to motivate myself.

My new job at Triad Group was also a more significant role than the one I'd held at Littler Savage. There, I'd found candidates for Rick and Craig's clients, period. But at Triad Group I was a "full desk" recruiter, which meant I had to open up my own clients and then find the candidates to fill those roles. I had never opened a new client myself before, so this would be new. (During my interview with Jim, when he'd asked me if I had opened up my own clients at Littler Savage, I'd lied and said yes, because I wanted the job so badly.)

Jim had mentioned during my interview that he liked to run his company like a law practice. He wanted to hire people with experience as a recruiter and a Rolodex full of candidates and clients. Triad Group was not the place for someone straight out of college or with minimal experience. There was no formal training on how to be a successful recruiter. You had your office and were on your own to build out your book of business. I got the job because Jim was impressed with the Silicon Valley companies I'd worked with and the roles I'd filled at those companies while at Littler Savage.

After the office manager set up my computer with Outlook, the applicant tracking system (ATS) Bullhorn, Dice, Hoovers, and all the interoffice files, she introduced me to the other recruiters. After meeting everyone, it was time for a cup of coffee.

As I entered the kitchen, I noticed a whiteboard with all the recruiters' names on it hung on the wall. There were eight recruiters in the company. Next to their name was their quota for the quarter. Next to their quota was how much they had billed for the quarter. Next to that number was how much they had billed for the year. Only two people had a number next to their name for how much they had billed for the quarter. The yearly figures for all eight recruiters were strikingly low; clearly, the tech-recruiting business was still enduring a sluggish period.

I walked back into my enormous office with my cup of coffee. I looked around my office, then took a deep breath and sat down at my desk.

When I'd first started recruiting, Donnita had expressed concern that my seizures might come back if I spent hours and hours staring at a computer screen. I'd also had those thoughts, and for the last few years I'd always made sure to take regular breaks and not focus for too long on words or images on my screen. Now that I'd been seizure-free for three years, though, I'd decided not to worry too much about staring at a computer screen anymore. I felt that I was one of the lucky ones—that my surgery had been a total success.

I was finding it difficult to be as positive about this new job as I was about my surgery. As I sat there at my desk that first day, some negative thoughts entered my mind: *Maybe I've bitten off more than I can chew. Maybe I should have found a recruiting job like my last one, where I only had to find candidates. In this climate, how am I going to find any new clients to open?*

CHAPTER 70

REALIZING THAT DECEMBER usually presented a lull in tech hiring, I was determined to secure at least one job to start working on before the year's end. Though I had never independently opened a client, I had observed Rick and Craig in action during their calls with potential new clients over the last couple of years. I drew inspiration from that.

Before even leaving for Seattle, I'd started two spreadsheets, one for companies and one for candidates. The "Company" spreadsheet contained a list of all the Bay Area companies Littler Savage had worked with, as well as all the software companies I'd tried to recruit people from. Next to each name, I'd listed the contacts I was able to find for each company. I started with the VPs, since they were easy to find on company websites. I found their emails by visiting the "News" page on their company website and scanning all the articles until I found the contact info for the PR person at the company. Once I found their email, I used the same email format for the VPs at the company.

The columns on my "Candidates" spreadsheet were labeled: *Name, Company, Position, Location,* and *Email.* I listed all the candidates I'd placed at Littler Savage, plus all candidates I'd spoken to and built a relationship with in the past.

Since I needed to find jobs to work on, I started with the "Company" spreadsheet. I thought about sending generic emails to the VPs on my list with my name, contact info, and information about the companies I had worked with and the roles I had filled, but instead I took a step back and decided to start by trying to send more targeted emails.

I logged on to Dice to see if any companies on my list had open roles; I noticed that a few were looking for software engineers. I had placed software engineers at Littler Savage but did not feel confident talking to candidates about their technical skills, so I moved on.

As I neared the end of my list, I noticed that one of my companies, a public software company in San Jose, was looking for a Senior Director of Product Marketing.

This was a company I had tried to recruit people from in the past; I also knew they partnered with BroadVision, our biggest client at Littler Savage. The job description mentioned that the role reported to the VP of Marketing. Since I had the email for the VP of Marketing, I decided to give it a shot.

I knew I would have only one shot at getting the VP's attention, so I took my time on the subject line for my email. I'd learned early on from Rick and Craig that these were the most important words I would put in my email. If you couldn't grab someone's attention with your subject, they likely wouldn't even open your email.

Since I had placed two VPs at BroadVision and BroadVision was a partner of this company, I decided to lead with that. *I PLACED SENIOR-LEVEL PEOPLE AT BROADVISION*, I wrote. Then, in the email itself, I wrote that I'd heard the VP was looking to add a Senior Director of Product Marketing to their team. (I didn't want to say that I'd seen the job on Dice; I wanted it to sound like I heard it from another source.) I said that I had placed two VPs at BroadVision; I listed some other Bay Area tech companies where I had placed people; and I mentioned that I had some great senior-level product marketers who were open to hearing about something new, and I would love to tell them about this opportunity. (I did have some great product marketers on my list, but I didn't know yet if they were open to hearing about something new. I figured I would find out if this VP expressed interest in working with me.)

I read and reread the email multiple times before I hit Send.

After sending that email—realizing that I didn't have the luxury of being picky about which jobs I would work on—I reached out to the VPs of engineering at the companies looking for software engineers. Then I moved on to sending more generic emails to all the other VPs at the companies on my list.

Since this last batch of companies did not have roles posted on their website or Dice, I figured I wouldn't hear back from them anytime soon; I just hoped they would remember my name when they needed to add someone to their team.

When I finally looked at the clock on my desk, I was surprised to see it was already 6:00 p.m.—time to go home. My first day at Triad Group was complete.

CHAPTER 71

TUESDAY AND WEDNESDAY, I kept tabs on new job postings on Dice and kept sending emails. When I arrived at the office on Thursday morning, an email from the VP of Marketing at the software company in San Jose was waiting for me.

In her email, the VP mentioned that she was still looking for that person to add to her team, and she asked if I had time to speak with her that day. I quickly responded that my afternoon was open, and we scheduled a call for 3:00 p.m.

Throughout the morning and early afternoon, my mind was preoccupied with thoughts of that 3:00 p.m. call. I was nervous; I had never dealt with a new client before. I knew I had to focus on the candidates I'd placed and the companies where I'd placed them during our call. Those results would help sell me as a good recruiter.

FINALLY, 3:00 P.M. rolled around—and the call went very well. I was nervous at the beginning, but once we got to talking, I relaxed. She said she was impressed with the companies I had worked with and the people I had placed. When she specifically mentioned BroadVision, I silently high-fived myself—my subject line had worked!

As our call drew to a close, she uttered the words I had been eagerly anticipating: "I would like to have you assist me with this role." Then, with a promise to send over a contract, she concluded the conversation.

As I hung up the phone, I did a double fist pump toward the ceiling, then jumped out of my chair and ran around my office like a little kid. It was a good thing I had my own office and the door was closed—I must have looked ridiculous. But I couldn't contain my excitement. My first client, in my first week!

Maybe this is the right job for me after all.

BE THERE WHEN I RETURN

— — —

Now THE HARD PART STARTED: I had to find good people to put in front of this VP.

I opened my "Candidates" spreadsheet and moved through the list, emailing every good product marketing candidate I found.

After sending the emails to the product marketing candidates, I created an email for the other candidates on my list. I told them I had just started a new job, mentioned that I was searching for a Senior Director of Product Marketing and asked if they knew any strong product marketers looking for a new job (I figured it was worth a shot; you never know who is connected to whom!), and asked them to keep me in mind if they were open to hearing about a new role or if their current company was doing any hiring.

After I finished those emails, I logged on to Dice to see if I could find any strong director-level product marketers. Since there were more people looking for jobs than there were companies looking to hire in tech at the moment, I was not surprised that I found some excellent candidates.

It felt like I was off to a good start. I'd planted the seeds; now I just had to wait and see what sprouted.

OVER THE NEXT few days, I heard back from a few people from my list who were interested in the role I'd emailed about; I also heard back from people I'd found on Dice. I set up calls with each one and screened them for the role. By the time I was done, I had six strong candidates to present to the VP of Marketing.

Over the next few weeks, a few of my candidates made it to the second and third round of interviews. I continued to look on Dice for companies with open roles and strong product marketing candidates.

DECEMBER ROLLED AROUND, and Jim told everyone that we'd be holding that year's Christmas party at Salish Lodge & Spa in Snoqualmie. I looked up the lodge: it was about thirty minutes from Bellevue and overlooked Snoqualmie Falls, a huge waterfall standing 286 feet—over 100 feet higher than Niagara Falls. I couldn't wait to see it.

A week before the party, the office manager, Debbie, walked into my office and handed me a piece of paper. "Jim had an idea for a fun contest at the party," she said. "We're having everyone write down a job they've had in the past that everyone else at the office will be surprised by. During the party, I'll hand everyone a piece of paper with all our names on one side of the paper and a list of jobs on the other. Whoever can match the most employees to their job will win a hundred-dollar gift certificate from the Salish Lodge & Spa."

"That is fun!" I said. "I'll have to think of a good one to write down."

"Great!" She smiled. "I'll be back at the end of the day to collect your piece of paper."

I deliberated for a while before settling on one specific job. I grinned as I wrote it down and discreetly folded the paper in half.

THE NIGHT OF THE Christmas party arrived. Jim had reserved one of the large private banquet rooms at the lodge. A large window on one of the walls overlooked the falls, which were lit up by spotlights. It was beautiful.

I introduced Donnita to my coworkers, and I got to meet their significant others. We enjoyed a great dinner, and after that it was time for our contest. Debbie explained the rules to the room, then handed out the piece of paper to everyone, along with a pen.

When I received my piece of paper, I placed it on the table in front of me. Of course, curiosity got the best of Donnita, and she looked down at the piece of paper and read what people had put down as their previous jobs.

"Really? *That* is what you put down?" She shook her head and smiled at me.

I laughed.

For my previous job, I'd written, *Worked at Chippendales.*

At forty-one years old, I was the youngest recruiter at Triad Group. Most recruiters were in their late forties or early fifties and had worked at the company for many years. I'd thought it would be funny to write down Chippendales—and I was right. The look on everyone's face when their eyes went down the paper and stopped at that line was priceless. Of course, everyone in the room knew it was me. And when the contest was over, we had a full-on Q&A session—everyone wanted to know what it had been like working at Chippendales.

As the year drew to a close, everything was falling into place. We loved our apartment in Kirkland, Natalie was adjusting to her new environment, Donnita liked her new role at The Cheesecake Factory, I felt good about my job, and I had gone another full year seizure-free.

I was hoping that 2002 would be the year that tech companies in the Bay Area would bounce back. I needed it to be; I'd only made $24,000 for the entire year. Something needed to change.

CHAPTER 72

THE NEW YEAR, 2002, started with promise: I noticed more companies were posting new job openings on Dice. The only problem was that thousands of people were looking for tech jobs in the Bay Area, and companies knew it. I continued to leave voice messages and emails with companies with open positions but kept getting the same response: *Sorry, I can't use an outside agency for any of my open roles. Maybe later in the year.*

In mid-January, I received an email from the VP of Marketing at the software company in San Jose I'd been working with. She said everyone liked my three remaining candidates, and they wanted them to come in the next week to do a forty-five-minute presentation in front of a few executives.

This was the first time a company had requested one of my candidates do a presentation. Even when I'd placed directors and VPs at BroadVision, they'd never asked for a presentation. But I did not think twice about it; I was just thrilled that I had three candidates going in for a final interview.

But then she gave me a less exciting piece of news: "Just so you know, we do have a fourth candidate scheduled to do a presentation as well."

My mouth dropped open. "Oh," I said. "Who is the other candidate?"

When she said his name, I was silent. I knew this guy; I had spoken to him while I worked at Littler Savage. I was mad at myself for not adding his name to my spreadsheet of candidates. *How could I forget to add his name to my spreadsheet?* I berated myself. He was one of the top product marketers in Silicon Valley. But he was currently a Senior Director of Product Marketing at Oracle; why would he want to leave that role for the same job at a smaller company?

"I know him," I said. "Is he really interested in leaving Oracle for a senior director role? I thought he was looking for a VP role."

"He is very interested in the role and has received high marks from everyone he has met," she said.

I didn't hold back. "If he wants the role, why are you having my candidates do a presentation?" I asked. "He's a stronger candidate than any of mine."

"We want more than one person to do a presentation," she said. "Anything can happen."

Sure it can, I thought.

The following week came and went, and my three candidates did their presentations—as did the candidate from Oracle. As expected, he got the job.

Next was the part of my job I hated: I had to tell my candidates that the company had gone with another candidate.

The first two conversations went well. They both mentioned that they'd spent a lot of time on the presentation, and of course they were disappointed that they hadn't gotten the job, but they didn't seem overly upset.

My third candidate, however, was livid. She started venting about how many hours she'd spent on the presentation. "I feel like I just gave them forty-five minutes of free consulting!" she complained.

I tried to calm her down, but she wasn't having it.

"I'm going to send the CEO a bill for two hours of consulting!" she snapped before we hung up.

After I got off the phone with her, I thought more about what she and the other two candidates had told me. They'd been asked to deliver very specific presentations. Were these the only four people to do presentations for the role? Had other people been asked to do presentations before these four had gone through those second and third round of interviews?

As the year went on, I heard from other people who'd had similar experiences during the interview process. I had also heard from people with many years of experience who applied for roles and never heard back from the company they'd applied to. Were companies posting jobs they were not actually hiring for, trying to build a list of top candidates for when they *were* ready to hire? Some people told me they'd gone through the entire interview process with a company, only to be told at the end of it that the role was on hold.

During this time, the companies were in a power position. Candidates needed jobs so badly that they were willing to give companies all their knowledge during interviews and presentations. I had no way of knowing the companies' intentions, but it sure felt like some of them were taking advantage of candidates.

Over the years, I have heard crazy stories from candidates about companies lying to them during the interview process—everything from lying about ARR (annual recurring revenue), burn rates, funding, pipelines, or key employees leaving to a CEO not telling a candidate that they'd hired a second person for the same role. Yes, you read that correctly: Someone told me a Series A company hired him to be their first VP of Marketing—and it was only on his first day, during a Zoom call with the CEO, when the CEO introduced "your co-VP of Marketing" and explained that he'd decided to hire *two* VPs of Marketing, one to run demand generation and the other person to run product marketing. The guy told me he just sat there in shock for a long moment and then resigned.

I still hear about stuff like that today. Some things never change. I wish they would.

As JANUARY CAME TO A CLOSE, my eyes rested on the calendar hanging beside my desk. I had circled an important date: Friday, February 1. It marked the last day I would receive my twice-monthly $1,500 draw; from then on, I would be on a 100 percent commission-based structure. The pressure was on; if I did not start making successful placements soon, our income would rely solely on Donnita's paycheck from The Cheesecake Factory, which came in at $13.50 an hour.

CHAPTER 73

OVER THE NEXT FEW MONTHS, getting companies in the Bay Area to let me work on their open roles was still challenging. I was lucky to have two companies give me a role to work on, but I knew I needed more than three to help pay the bills.

Even though it was tough to get hiring managers at companies to give me roles to work on, I continued contacting hiring managers at tech companies in Silicon Valley. I was building a robust database of director- and VP-level hiring managers. I knew hiring had to start picking up again at some point. The million-dollar question was . . . *when*?

I was putting good candidates in front of hiring managers, but my candidates kept coming in at second place. The companies would never tell me if the reason they'd decided not to go with my candidate was because there was a fee associated with that choice, but it sure felt like that was happening.

IN JUNE, TRIAD GROUP moved into a new office—a space in downtown Bellevue, located on the sixteenth floor of a building on the corner of NE 8th Street and 110th Avenue NE.

The new office was much nicer than our previous office. Eight offices faced west, with large windows overlooking Bellevue, Lake Washington, and downtown Seattle. There was a big corner office—Jim's office—with views to the west and Mount Rainer in the south. There were also four offices across the hall from the offices with views that had large floor-to-ceiling glass so you could see who was in their office working (and who wasn't). No one wanted to be in those offices.

There were eight recruiters at Triad Group at this point, so everyone was going to be able to get an office with a view. Jim decided to let the top billers pick out the office they wanted first. Since I was the low man on the totem pole, I didn't get to pick an office; I got stuck with the last one available. My office was the smallest and was located next to Jim's large corner office. The view was nice, but my desk faced a wall, with the window behind me.

So far, 2002 wasn't working out so well for me.

As JULY DREW NEARER and my one-year anniversary at Triad Group approached, the reality that I had not yet made a single placement weighed heavily on me. Doubts started to creep in, and I began questioning whether recruiting was the right career for me. Perhaps this industry wasn't a good fit; had I made a mistake pursuing this path?

As the financial pressure mounted, I began considering finding a bartending job at night to supplement my income and help pay the bills. The challenge was that I had no bar or restaurant connections in the Seattle area.

I decided to stop by a few bars and restaurants in Kirkland and Bellevue to see if they were looking to hire. There were no openings. But one day, Donnita came home from work and told me that a guy she'd worked with at The Cheesecake Factory was now the manager at a new restaurant/bar called Tap House that was about to open in downtown Bellevue.

"I told him about all your bartending experience," she said, handing me his card. "He's expecting your call."

I was grateful to Donnita for making the connection, but I hesitated to call the guy; I didn't really want to return to bartending. But we needed the money, so the next day, I called.

I MET STEVE at the Tap House a few days later, and he gave me a tour of the place. It was a cool concept. The menu looked great, and they had 160 beers on tap.

"Donnita told me about all the places you've bartended," he said. "Impressive!"

"Thanks," I said. "Yeah, I've spent a lot of time pouring drinks in my life."

"Sounds like it," he said. "Unfortunately, we do have a full staff of bartenders right now—but you never know when something will open up. I'll definitely give you a call when that happens!"

"Please do," I said, not at all disappointed. Bartending was something I felt ready to leave in the past. I decided not to give up on recruiting. *I'm going to make this work*, I promised myself.

— — —

DONNITA WAS STARTING to feel overwhelmed by the reality of all of us living on her hourly wage at The Cheesecake Factory. She was starting to feel like things might never get better.

"I drive around neighborhoods and go to open houses sometimes," she admitted, "and when I do, all I can think is *We are never going to be able to buy a house.*"

We were relying on credit cards to cover a significant portion of our expenses, and our debt was accumulating. Between our credit card and medical bills, we now owed a whopping $50,000—and since we could only make the minimum payment on our credit cards, we were getting killed by the high interest rates. At this rate, we were never going to be able to pay off our credit cards.

Unfortunately for us, the next four months did not get much better. As November started, I still had not made a placement.

CHAPTER 74

A FEW DAYS LATER, a glimmer of hope appeared in my inbox as I received an email from the VP of HR at BroadVision—one of the many VPs I'd reached out to in recent months. *We're looking for a Director of Corporate Communications*, she wrote. *Would you be interested in helping fill the role?*

The timing could not have been better. This was the first time a company had contacted me proactively, asking for my help filling an open role. It felt like a good omen.

Then I got to the part of the email where she mentioned a placement fee for the role. *If you do place the role*, she said, *we can only pay a flat fee of $10,000.*

My placement fees were usually between 15 percent and 20 percent of the base salary. A role like this would have a base salary between $130K and $150K—so with this flat fee, I'd be getting less than half (possibly way less than half) of my normal fee. After paying off a portion of my draw and taxes, I would only clear around $1,000.

But I was not in a position to say no. I wrote back and said I was interested in working on the role, and a flat fee of $10,000 would be acceptable.

Better than nothing, I thought.

WITHIN A WEEK, I found four good people for the BroadVision role. Their hiring manager liked three of them, and she got them going on the interview process.

It was now the beginning of December, and the end of the year was quickly approaching. The hiring manager wanted to put one of my candidates in front of a group of people.

"Will he need to do a presentation?" I asked.

"No," she said.

Small victories; I was happy about that.

"We hope to finish the interview process by the end of the year," she said, "but it's tricky around the holidays—there's a chance it might roll into January."

I crossed my fingers, along with anything else I could think of on my body that I could cross. I needed this placement to happen, even if I would only clear $1,000.

DECEMBER ARRIVED, and it brought with it year-end reviews. Jim sent out an email outlining the schedule for our one-on-one reviews. The purpose was to reflect on our achievements in 2002 and discuss our plans for the upcoming year.

My meeting with Jim was scheduled for Friday at 3:00 p.m.

Despite having two candidates in the interviewing process with different companies and a highly promising candidate in the works for BroadVision, I could not escape the fact that I hadn't made a single placement since joining Triad Group. Would this year-end review be the end for me?

CHAPTER 75

I SAT DOWN AT THE dining room table with Donnita and Natalie. Donnita placed a plate of chicken marsala in front of me. It looked amazing. The chicken breast was lightly browned and cooked perfectly, and it sat on a bed of al dente pasta with mushrooms. The aroma of the marsala sauce filled the room. Donnita topped the dish off with a sprinkle of fresh parsley.

"This looks amazing!" I said.

Donnita's face brightened. "Thank you! Dig in."

Her culinary skills were truly remarkable. Each evening, she treated us to a delightful and unique meal. Her cooking was so exquisite that I frequently boasted to my coworkers, claiming I had dined at a fantastic new restaurant in Kirkland the previous night. When they inquired about the restaurant's name, I would playfully respond with "The Donnita Café."

After we finished dinner, I had my usual: a Baileys coffee and a chocolate-covered almond biscotti.

Donnita could tell something was on my mind as I dunked my biscotti into my coffee.

"What's on your mind?" she asked.

I stared into my coffee. "I have a feeling that Jim is going to fire me tomorrow."

Donnita wasn't expecting that; I felt her body tense next to mine. "Why? Did Jim tell you that?"

"No, but I haven't made a single placement since I started working there," I said morosely.

"I know, but you said you got close to placing some people but the companies picked other candidates," she said. "And don't you have a candidate that a company really likes right now?"

"Yes," I said. "But that doesn't mean anything right now."

I reached into my pocket and pulled out a piece of paper. I unfolded it and placed it on the table. "Jim sent this out to everyone a few days ago," I said, pushing it toward Donnita.

She picked it up and read it.

The last line caught her attention, as it had mine:

This is a sales organization. If you do not produce, you will be replaced.

CHAPTER 76

FRIDAY MORNING, I woke up with a feeling of unease deep in the pit of my stomach as I made my way down the hall to the kitchen. Donnita was busy making breakfast for herself and Natalie as I squeezed around her, reached into a cabinet, and grabbed a bowl.

As I ate my Honey Nut Cheerios with banana, I could not stop thinking about my meeting with Jim later that afternoon. I started questioning every decision I had made, doubting my abilities as a recruiter. I knew I had given 100 percent—but apparently, that wasn't enough.

I also knew I was not the only person having a bad year. People in the office who had been top billers the previous year were having the worst year of their careers. Unfortunately, I was the only one with a big fat zero next to their name for Q4 and yearly billings.

Usually, when I ate my cereal in the morning, Donnita would walk up behind me and say, "Slow down! You don't need to inhale it."

This morning, she did not need to say a word as I picked through my cereal and finally lifted my spoon to my mouth. Each bite I took felt like a small pause in the whirlwind of thoughts and worries.

I could not eat any more cereal. I got up from the table, emptied my bowl down the drain, cleaned the bowl, and placed it in the dishwasher. I walked into the bathroom, nervously brushed my teeth, and shaved my face. I turned on the hot water and wiped down my face. I moved closer to the mirror, staring intensely into it.

Donnita walked into the bathroom, moved behind me, and wrapped her arms around me.

"I know you're nervous about your meeting," she said gently. "But everything is going to be okay."

I continued staring into the mirror. "What am I going to do if Jim fires me?"

"If that happens, we will figure something out. You need to stay positive."

I took a deep breath and moved back from the mirror. "I know. I'm trying."

She squeezed me, and kissed me on the cheek. "I love you."

"I love you," I said, never more grateful for her support.

As I exited the bathroom and went down the hallway, I spotted Natalie sitting at the kitchen table. I leaned over and planted a kiss on her cheek. "Bye, sweetie." I grabbed my keys from the counter and headed toward the front door.

"I love you, Dad! Have a great day!" my little girl yelled after me.

I stopped turning the door handle and turned back toward her with a big smile. "Thank you! I love you too."

I opened the door and walked out.

CHAPTER 77

I ENCOUNTERED AN UNEXPECTED traffic jam as I merged onto the I-405 South. Frustration crept in. *Of all days, why today?*

The standstill seemed to last forever, but eventually the traffic began to inch forward.

After what felt like an eternity, I finally reached the NE 8th Street exit and entered the garage. I was not late.

As I stepped into the office, I immediately sensed a tense atmosphere. Evidently, I was not the only one who had experienced a sleepless night. On my way to the kitchen to get my coffee, I could not help but notice people huddled together, exchanging whispers and casting glances in my direction. I could almost feel their apprehension and was sure they believed that Jim might be considering letting me go.

As I stirred the creamer into my coffee, I glanced at the two large whiteboards on the wall. One board showed the placements that had been made for the month. The second board showed what each recruiter had billed for the quarter and the year. There I was on the bottom.

I made my way back to my office and got to work. Time seemed to stretch on endlessly. I kept checking the clock on my desk. I needed to stay focused.

A day earlier, I'd emailed Jim a list of the people I had in the interview process, details on my business that year, and what I was projecting for next year.

The clock on my desk read 1:00 p.m. I walked into the kitchen and grabbed my lunch. Donnita had made me a turkey-and-Swiss sandwich and put in a bag of Fritos corn chips and a small Tupperware container of mixed fruit. I ate my lunch at my desk, working to distract myself.

About thirty minutes later, an email came in from the hiring manager at one of the companies where I had a candidate in second-round interviews:

Michael, I wanted to let you know that we have decided to move forward with an offer to another candidate for the Director of Product Marketing role. Can you please tell Paul that everyone enjoyed meeting him? Thank you. — Al

I was not surprised that they'd chosen someone else, but I'd been hoping against hope that my candidate would get the offer.

Oh well. I had to keep moving forward.

About an hour later, I received another email—this one from the other candidate I had in a second-round interview with another company:

Michael, thank you for putting me in front of Comergent. I really enjoyed speaking with everyone, but I have decided to take an offer from a larger public software company. Thank you again for all of your help. — Dave

Could my day be going any worse?

I looked at the clock on my desk. It read 2:59 p.m.

Time to face the music.

THE WALK TO Jim's office felt like a never-ending journey, with each step growing heavier and more foreboding. As I got closer to his office, my stomach started to tighten, and I had this strange feeling throughout my entire body, similar to when I stood on the roof of my apartment in LA. The only difference this time was that if something terrible happened, it would affect *two* other people besides me—Donnita and Natalie.

I lingered outside Jim's door and noticed he was on the phone. After a moment, he waved me into his office.

"Close the door," he said softly, his hand over the phone receiver.

I gently shut the door behind me and nervously settled into one of the chairs in front of his large oak desk. My palms felt clammy and my heart raced with anticipation. While Jim wrapped up his call, I sought solace by gazing out the expansive floor-to-ceiling window, taking in the captivating view of the Seattle skyline.

Jim finally got off the phone, and our meeting began.

With a deep breath, I composed myself and calmly shared a detailed account of my year's experiences with Jim. I honestly discussed the challenges I'd faced, particularly in finding companies willing to pay a fee for my services. I explained that I had come close to making placements on several occasions, but ultimately the companies had either chosen another candidate or my candidates had accepted other offers. I knew I was not the only person in the office telling him this story.

Jim picked up a piece of paper from his desk. It was the list of people I had in the interview process. "It looks like you have three people in the interview process right now—two in the second round and one in the final round," he said. "How many of these people do you think you will be able to place?"

"Well, when I sent you that yesterday, I did have three people in the interview process," I said honestly. "But in the last few hours, I lost two of them. I got an email from one candidate letting me know that he took another offer, and one from the other client letting me know that they made another candidate an offer and they accepted."

"Okay . . . so then you only have the person interviewing at BroadVision, right?"

"Correct." I sat up taller in my chair. "But I feel strongly that they will make him an offer and he will accept!"

Jim leaned back in his chair.

In an effort to shift the conversation, I brought up my observations regarding a positive change in companies' openness to paying fees to external recruiters. I emphasized that during my time at Triad Group, I had diligently built a substantial database of hiring managers and potential candidates with impressive backgrounds. Additionally, I highlighted the efforts I had made to foster relationships with hiring managers, many of whom had expressed their intention to offer me roles to work on in the upcoming year's Q1.

Despite trying to convey my optimism for a successful 2003, I could not shake the nagging thought that Jim might still decide to let me go.

What the hell am I going to do if he fires me? Why the hell did I think I could pull this off? Maybe we should have just stayed in LA.

I steeled myself, ready to hear the words I had dreaded all along.

Jim listened quietly, absorbing the information thoughtfully. He then placed his palms on the back of his head and leaned back in his chair. "I understand it's been a challenging year for you," he acknowledged. "You're not alone in facing difficulties; others in the office have also faced challenges. And, truth be told, it's been tough for me as an owner these past few years."

His words struck a chord, and I felt a mix of relief and empathy knowing that my colleagues were experiencing struggles similar to mine. Still, I could not help but wonder about the outcome of our conversation. The uncertainty continued to weigh on my mind as I listened to what Jim had to say next.

"I've listened to you on the phone," he continued, "and I must say, I like how you talk to people. Your work ethic is commendable, and I believe success as a recruiter is within your reach. You just need a little luck. I genuinely think you have all the necessary qualities to thrive in this role. I believe you will do very well here."

His encouraging words gave me a glimmer of hope. Relief and gratitude flooded through me; it was a moment of validation and reassurance. I was expecting words of disappointment and termination, not praise. I realized that my efforts and determination had not gone unnoticed by my boss.

I mustered the courage to speak, my voice shaky. "Thank you. I . . . I thought you were going to fire me."

Jim leaned forward in his chair. "Not a chance. I really hope that Broad-Vision placement happens for you. Thank you for coming in, Michael."

I slowly got up from my chair. "Thank you, that means a lot to me."

I left our meeting with a newfound sense of motivation, ready to embrace the upcoming challenges with renewed optimism.

THE FIRST THING I did when I sat back down at my desk was pick up my phone and call Donnita.

It rang . . . and rang . . . and rang.

Then, finally: "Hello?"

"I still have a job!" I said, my voice cracking.

"I told you he wasn't going to fire you," she exclaimed. "What did he say?"

I leaned back in my chair. "He said that he believes I have all the qualities to be a great recruiter and that all I need is a little luck."

"Good," she said. "I agree with Jim. I think you are going to be a great recruiter. You have already proven that you can do this job."

I looked up at the ceiling, trying to collect my emotions. Exhaling slowly, I said, "I know. I know. I have to go. I just wanted to let you know that everything worked out. I love you. I'll see you at home."

"I love you!"

With renewed determination, I sat back up in my chair and refocused on my work. The belief that Jim had in me motivated me even further. I knew I had to prove to him and myself that his decision not to let me go was the right one.

CHAPTER 78

ON MONDAY, JANUARY 6, I received an email from my candidate who'd been interviewing at BroadVision.

I was afraid to open it. Why hadn't he accepted the offer on Friday? Had he decided to reject it?

I finally clicked on the email, which was short and sweet:

Michael, I wanted to let you know that I accepted the offer from BroadVision. I start on Monday the fifteenth. Thank you again for all of your help.

AFTER THE VP of HR at BroadVision called to let me know she had received the signed offer letter, I jumped out of my chair, strode to the kitchen, and wrote my placement on the whiteboard. Since the month had just started, it was the first one for Q1 2003. A few coworkers congratulated me as I put my achievement on the board, filled with pride—and relief.

On March 14, I made my second placement. Things were looking up—but I had a ways to climb. As Q1 ended, I was still positioned at the bottom of the board for total billings for the quarter.

CHAPTER 79

IT WAS EARLY afternoon on March 31 when the email came into my inbox. The email was from a guy named Alex, who said he was a product marketer with a San Jose company called Callidus Software. He said someone had referred him to me, and he was starting to look for something new. He asked if I was open to having a conversation with him.

I had never heard of Callidus Software, but of course I was open to talking. I replied to his email, and we set up a call.

WHEN I SPOKE with Alex a couple of days later, we discussed what type of role he was interested in and what size company he would be interested in working for. After he filled me in, he decided it was time to change the subject.

"I have a feeling that my boss is going to get fired," he told me.

I blinked. His boss was the VP of Marketing—a big role. "Really? Why?"

"He and the CEO don't see eye to eye on some things," he said. "You might want to drop an email to the CEO."

"Can I get the CEO's email from you?"

He was happy to give it; I wrote it down, and soon afterward we said our goodbyes.

After I got off the phone, I pulled up the Callidus Software website and researched the company, the CEO, and the other executives, including the VP of Marketing. After doing some research, I started to craft an email to the CEO.

Once the email itself was written, I knew I had to put something in the subject line that would catch his eye. I played with many different phrases before finally settling on *I HEARD YOU ARE LOOKING FOR A VP OF MARKETING.*

Considering the fact that he hadn't even fired the current one yet, I figured that should get his attention.

BE THERE WHEN I RETURN

- - -

THREE DAYS LATER, I received a reply. He said he was indeed looking for a VP of Marketing, and suggested that we set up a time to speak on the phone about the search.

I read the email repeatedly to ensure I read it correctly, then quietly celebrated my win. *It worked!*

AFTER ONE PHONE call, the CEO said he wanted me to work on the search for his new VP of Marketing . He'd said the company was positioned to have an IPO by the end of the year, so I felt I could probably ask for a retainer—but before I could even utter the word, he jumped in and said he did not want to do a retainer.

"If you're okay doing the search on a contingency basis, I want you on it," he said.

I paused briefly and weighed my options. I would still get a significant placement fee if I found his person. "Okay," I agreed, "a contingency basis is fine."

"I can only do twenty percent of the base salary," he said in a tone that left no room for negotiation.

I'd hoped the percentage would be higher, but 20 percent wasn't bad. "Okay," I said. "I'm okay with that."

"Great!" he said. "I'll have HR send over a contract by the end of the day."

After I hung up the phone, I was almost beside myself with excitement. *I have my first VP of Marketing search.* I definitely hadn't seen this one coming.

WE SIGNED THE contract a few days later, and I was off to the races. I contacted every VP of Marketing I knew and asked them if they were open to hearing about something new—or knew anyone who might be. Over the next few weeks, I found a few decent candidates. Then, one day, I received an email from an interested person who was the VP of Worldwide Marketing at NetManage, a software company based in Cupertino, California.

We spoke a few days later. I liked the guy's background and thought he could be a fit for what the CEO at Callidus was looking for. The candidate also liked what he was hearing from me about Callidus; he asked me to put him in front of the CEO.

After my candidate met the CEO, he moved quickly through the interview process. On May 12, he accepted their offer. He would start in June.

Finally, things were starting to happen for me. That same month, I made two other placements. My goal for 2003 had been to make at least one placement a month. As May ended, I was up to five placements for the year. I was on track.

For the first time since starting at Triad Group, I felt that the recruiting business might work out for me after all.

I had no idea what was in store for me in the next four months.

CHAPTER 80

"Have you heard of LinkedIn?"

I was on the phone with Rich, a product marketer I had known for a few years, just chatting. As always, I was a sponge ready to soak up knowledge. "No," I said. "What is it?"

"A new social media site," he said.

"Really? Another one?" Maybe they were looking to hire some people. "I've checked out Friendster and Myspace; I'm not a big social media fan."

He gauged my disdain from the tone of my voice. "This is different," he insisted. "You need to check it out. Here, do it right now—go to www.linkedin.com."

I decided to give it a shot; I played along and went to the website. "Okay, now what?"

"I'll give you my login and password and explain why it's so different from other social media sites. I'll change my password when we get off the phone, so don't get any ideas," he joked.

"Okay, let's do it."

Once I logged in, Rich walked me through how to find people.

"Under 'location,' put in a zip code, and under 'company,' put a company of your choice—then hit Search," he said.

I did what he said, then sat there and watched as profiles of people populated my screen—profiles with tons of information, including where they worked, their name, their location, and their job title.

"Holy shit!"

He could tell I was impressed. "I told you! You can also search by title. Should make it easier to find the roles you are recruiting for."

I thought back to my days at Littler Savage, when all I'd had were directories of random names at companies, with no clue what their job title was. Now, I could focus specifically on the positions I wanted to fill, and I would know who the people were.

"And that's only people at one company," Rich said. "Imagine getting all that info from other tech companies in the Bay Area!"

I still wasn't entirely sure how all this worked. "But this is your account; will I be able to see the same people when I open an account?"

"Yep! Once you set up your profile, you'll need to send me an invite to connect with you. Once I accept your invite, you can see the profiles of people I'm connected with and those who are a second connection to you. Everyone in Silicon Valley is signing up."

"Wow." I shook my head with wonder at all the possibilities this was going to open up for me. "How much does this cost?"

"It's free for now."

We hung up, and I got to work opening up a LinkedIn account.

I MADE SOME strategic decisions while filling out my profile on LinkedIn. When I got to the location section, I took a step back and thought it through. If I put a Seattle zip code, people might pigeonhole me—think I only knew people in Seattle and only worked with companies in the area. Since all my contacts and clients were in the Bay Area, I elected to use the zip code for Redwood Shores instead.

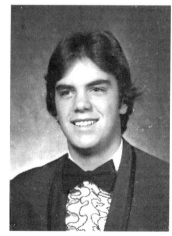

When I added my education information, I added St. Mary's College of California, bachelor's degree, Business Administration/Economics. I decided not to add Cañada Junior College, but I did add St. Ignatius College Prep—I thought the fact that I'd graduated from one of the top private high schools in San Francisco would add value to my profile. (Thank you again, Patty Martin!)

The other thing I decided to do was leave my age off my profile altogether. I omitted graduation dates from St. Mary's

St Ignatius –
Senior Year - 1978

and St. Ignatius, and all the jobs I'd had before Littler Savage. I didn't want to fill my profile with a bunch of bartending jobs. So, looking at my

LinkedIn profile, you might conclude that I'd graduated from college in 1998 and my first job was at Littler Savage.

I was all ready to go. I sent a connection request to Rich, and he accepted.

Since I saw so many people from Siebel Systems on LinkedIn, I decided to start off by sending connection requests to people in marketing and sales roles. I liked trying to pull people from Siebel because they hired top talent, especially people with MBAs from top schools. They also had a great training program. I always felt that if someone at Siebel was open to looking at something new, I could place them.

I was amazed by how quickly people responded to connect with me. Once they accepted my connection request, I asked them for their work email so we could stay in touch. One person got back to me with their work email—and bam, I was all set! Now I knew the email format at Siebel.

After that worked so efficiently, I went through my list of other top tech companies in the Bay Area and sent every marketer and salesperson I could find a connection request.

By a few weeks later, I'd built a strong database of candidates in the Bay Area—and I had all their work emails too. I could now email a potential candidate to see if they were open to hearing about something new, and I could also email the hiring manager at a company if they had open roles. Going forward, anytime I got someone new on the phone, I always ended the conversation with "Can I send you a LinkedIn connection request?"

CHAPTER 81

MY CANDIDATE STARTED his new role at Callidus in June 2003. I knew they would be hiring more people soon, since they were getting ready for an IPO later in the year, so I spent some time strategizing about how to get in on the action. After some consideration, I decided to ask my recently placed candidate to introduce me to the head of HR at Callidus—but before I could do that, I received a call from the head of HR at Callidus.

During our call, she congratulated me on finding their VP of Marketing, then asked, "Do you only place executives, or do you work on other roles?"

"What roles do you have open?" I asked.

"Lots," she said.

We discussed the open roles and decided I would help on six of them: two directors of business development/alliances, one director of product management, two software engineers, and one account executive in New York.

During this time, there were still a lot of companies that had not recovered from the Dot Bomb and 9/11. I was fortunate that Callidus was one of the companies that was growing.

Now I just had to find some candidates.

As JULY APPROACHED, I had multiple candidates in the final interview process for all the open roles. By the time July ended, I had placed six people at Callidus, including three in one day. I also signed up a new client on a retainer.

After I put my final placement in July on the whiteboard, some coworkers came into my office to congratulate me on having a monster July. One of them was Dorothy, a longtime Triad Group employee who'd seen first-hand the struggles I'd experienced in 2002.

"Congratulations, Michael," she said with a big smile. "You deserve all the success. I must tell you, I'm impressed with how humble you are. A few people in the office would be handling this success differently."

I ducked my head and smiled back at her. "Thank you."

Even as a kid, I was never the person who flaunted when he did something well. I learned early in life that confidence is silent, and insecurities are loud. In our boastful social media era, it's tough for many people to remain humble. There are also a lot of people who stretch the truth about their success. When I was living in LA, I learned to believe only 10 percent of what people (especially people I met at bars and nightclubs) told me until I learned more about them. As social media rose in popularity and I saw so many people posting constantly about how successful they were, I decided to bring that rule back.

I'D SET A TRIAD GROUP company record in July for the largest monthly billings ever, so at the beginning of August, Jim emailed the office that he'd set up a lunch at Daniel's Broiler, a high-end steak house on the twenty-first floor of the Bank of America building in downtown Bellevue.

I popped over to Jim's office when I saw his email. "Thank you so much for offering to celebrate my accomplishments with this lunch," I said.

"You deserve it!" Jim said. "You're a great example of perseverance."

"I really appreciate that," I said. "But I'm a little uncomfortable with all these accolades . . . You know how quickly things can change in this crazy world."

"That's true," Jim said, "but you've worked hard, and we need to celebrate your accomplishment. It doesn't matter what happens tomorrow."

I finally gave in. "Okay," I said. "I'll be there."

"HOW WAS YOUR big lunch?" Donnita asked when I got home from work that evening.

Jim had made me stand up and tell everyone at lunch the story of my time at Triad Group. I'd explained to them how until this previous month, I'd had terrible luck since starting this job, but I'd just kept grinding because I'd known my luck would eventually change. At the end of the day, I'd told them, the only thing we can do is keep moving forward. And I'd meant everything I said. But it had felt awkward being in the spotlight like that.

"It was fine," I said, shrugging.

She knew I was not excited about being put up on a pedestal. "I'm glad you told Jim you would go to the lunch," she said. "You deserve it. You worked hard for everything that is happening right now."

I wrapped her in my arms and kissed her, "I really feel like things are finally coming together."

As I held Donnita close, a whirlwind of thoughts flew through my mind. I was planning to ask Jim a favor on Monday morning—and when I thought about how he might respond to my request, my heart filled with apprehension.

CHAPTER 82

On Monday morning, I stood at the entrance of Jim's office. His face hovered just inches from his monitor, alternating between scanning a paper on his desk and glancing back at the screen. Upon noticing my presence in his office, he promptly pushed himself back in his chair and offered me a smile. "Morning!" he said.

"Morning," I said hesitantly. "Do you have a minute?"

"Sure."

I turned, shut his door, and sat down across from him. "How was your weekend?

"Good, how about you?" he asked.

"We went to Alki Beach on Saturday. It was fun."

I pulled out a piece of paper, placed it on his desk, and slid it toward him.

He picked it up. "What's this?"

"I wanted to ask if you are comfortable paying me my commission in advance," I blurted out. "All the money from Callidus will come in two months if they pay the invoice on time. I've listed all my placements and my total commission. Would you be okay paying me the total over the next four paychecks?"

Jim leaned back in his chair and looked over the numbers on the paper. Then he sat up in his chair. "Have all the candidates you placed started working at Callidus?"

I was really hoping that he would not ask me that question. "Two of them have given notice and are planning on starting next week."

He leaned back in his chair and started to rock forward and back slowly. "Why do you need the money now?"

"I want to surprise Donnita with something."

He looked down at the paper again. "Okay. I can split the commission up over the next four pay periods. You'll get the first check this Friday."

"Thank you," I exclaimed. "Thank you!"

Jim handed me the piece of paper. I got up from my chair.

"Thank you," I said again. "This means a lot to me."

"You're welcome."

I practically skipped back down the hallway to my office; I was so thrilled that Jim was open to paying me in advance. Still, I couldn't stop thinking about the three things that must happen for all this to work out: First, the candidate must show up on the first day of work—and I still had two candidates who hadn't started yet. Second, the candidate must stay employed through the guarantee period—at Callidus, that was sixty days. And finally, the company had to pay the invoice.

I sat down at my desk, got back to work, and tried not to think about what would happen if the six people I'd placed at Callidus didn't complete the first two items on the list.

CHAPTER 83

WHEN I ARRIVED HOME from work on Friday, I found Donnita preparing what was sure to be another amazing dinner. I planted a gentle kiss on her cheek, went to our bedroom to change out of my work clothes and into a pair of sweatpants and a T-shirt, and then strolled down the hallway to Natalie's room to say hi.

Natalie was jumping up and down on her bed, acting out scenes from the movie *Toy Story*, so she didn't notice me standing there at first. But when she did, she yelled, "Daddy!" and ran to me.

I knelt down and gave her a big hug.

"Did you have a good day at work?" she asked as she ran back to her bed and continued jumping up and down on it.

"Yes, I did," I said. "How was your day?"

"Fun. We played basketball today. I like basketball."

"Dinner should be ready soon," I said.

"Okay."

I left Natalie's room and made my way back to the kitchen, where Donnita was putting the finishing touches on dinner.

"Dinner is ready," she said. "Let's sit down."

"Hold on," I said. "I have something you need to look at."

"Can't it wait until after dinner?"

"Not really."

When she wasn't looking, I reached into the pocket of my sweatpants, pulled out an envelope, and placed it on the plate in front of the chair where she usually sat for dinner.

When she walked toward me, I pointed to the envelope on her plate. "You need to open that."

She tilted her head. "What is it?"

"Open it."

Donnita's expression shifted from confusion to a smile as she gazed at me, her curiosity piqued. With a swift motion, she reached over, delicately picked up the envelope, and opened it. She pulled the paper out of the envelope, and her gaze shifted from the words on the paper, back to me, and then back to the paper.

"What is this?" she asked.

"It's my paycheck."

"Why is your paycheck so big?"

"Jim is advancing my commission over the next four pay periods. There will be three more checks that big."

"What?" Her eyes widened.

"Yep!" I had a Cheshire Cat grin on my face.

Donnita threw her arms around me. "Congratulations. You deserve everything that is happening to you."

"I thought with the money that's coming in we could pay off some of our debt and"—I drew out a long pause for dramatic effect—"BUY A HOUSE!"

"What?" Donnita's hands flew up to her mouth. "Really?"

Natalie came running into the kitchen. "What's going on?"

"We are going to go buy a *house!*" Donnita exclaimed.

It was the perfect moment for a big group hug.

CHAPTER 84

In October, we moved into our new house in Issaquah, twelve miles east of Bellevue. With its large evergreen trees, greenery, and sizable lake, Issaquah feels like you are up in the mountains, but you are only seventeen miles from Seattle.

The process of finding our house was a bit stressful, but we were lucky to find one that we liked in a neighborhood we loved.

The most interesting part of the process was the surprise we'd gotten at the title company.

Donnita and I were thrilled to be signing off on our new house as we drove to the title company in Bellevue. We sat at the table with the title company representative as she started to go through all the paperwork that needed our initials and signatures.

She handed us pens. "Congratulations!"

"Thank you!" we said in stereo.

As Donnita and I started to go through the documents, adding our initials at the places pointed out by the title representative, Donnita noticed that I wasn't moving and my eyes were glued to one of the pages, even though I had already added my initials. The title representative was ready to turn to the next page but noticed I was still looking down at the document. She looked over at Donnita.

"Michael!" Donnita called out. Even though I'd been seizure-free for six years, she still kept an eye on me, and she knew that one of my triggers was when I stared at an object for a prolonged period.

I didn't answer; I just continued staring at the document that I had just initialed.

The title rep glanced back at Donnita and then back at me.

"Michael!"

This time, Donnita's voice got my attention, and I looked right at her.

"Are you okay?" she asked.

"I'm fine," I reassured her. "Sorry. I just still can't believe we are sitting here about to buy a house."

The title representative flipped the page and pointed to a section at the bottom that needed our initials. We were about six or seven pages into the documents when she said excitedly, "Wow, you guys got a great deal on your mortgage."

I was a bit thrown off by her comment. The loan officer from Washington Mutual had told us we were getting a five-year adjustable-rate mortgage at 4.25 percent. I thought it was okay but nothing spectacular, so the comment seemed out of place. "A five-year ARM at 4.25 percent?" I said. "I didn't know it was that great of a deal."

She froze; then she grabbed the paperwork and flipped to the document's first page, which had our mortgage terms. She pointed to a line with her pen. "You guys have a thirty-year fixed mortgage at 4.25 percent, not a five-year ARM. It looks like someone made a little mistake."

She spun the document around to show us. There it was: 360 payments at 4.25 percent.

Donnita and I just looked at each other. We didn't know what to say.

"A thirty-year fixed should be 6.15 percent—you guys just hit the lottery," she said.

Donnita smiled, looked at me, and said, "Just keep signing."

"Will someone see this and change it back to a five-year ARM?" I asked.

"I doubt it," the woman said. "An underwriter already reviewed this paperwork; once we're done signing here, it will go to County Records. I can call you tomorrow to confirm everything's gone through as it should, if you like."

"That would be great," I said.

We finished signing the documents and then drove back to our apartment in Kirkland.

I didn't sleep much that night. I had all these crazy dreams about getting a call from the woman at the title company telling us the bank had caught their mistake, and the mortgage terms were being changed back to the original five-year ARM at 4.25 percent.

- - -

THE NEXT DAY, the woman called.

"How does it all look?" I asked cautiously.

"Great!" she said. "Your mortgage is a thirty-year fixed at 4.25 percent."

"Oh wow," I said. "Thank you!"

"Congratulations!" she said.

Donnita and I realized how blessed we were not to have that five-year ARM mortgage a few years later, when the housing market crashed. When home prices declined steeply after peaking in mid-2006, it became more difficult for borrowers to refinance their loans, and the ARM mortgages began to reset at higher interest rates (causing higher monthly payments). Some people we knew who had five-year ARM mortgages lost their homes because they could not pay the higher mortgage payment. That could have easily been us.

AS 2003 DREW TO A CLOSE, all the pieces fell into place. The year had been transformative, and I was elated to have made five more successful placements at Callidus Software in the latter half of the year, bringing my total to an impressive sixteen placements for the year. Equally significant was the milestone of completing my sixth year seizure-free, a reminder of the strength and resilience I had developed in facing life's challenges.

With so many positive developments in my professional and personal life, I couldn't help but reflect on my journey over the last year. The memory of that unsettling day when I feared losing my job was still vivid, but it served as a poignant reminder of how rapidly circumstances can change—and how good my life was right now.

CHAPTER 85

IT WAS JANUARY 2004, my first day back in the office to start the new year. I logged into LinkedIn and noticed that they had added a new feature to people's profiles called "Recommendations." I could now ask people to leave a recommendation on the quality of my work. I immediately emailed all the VPs at Callidus to see if they would leave me a recommendation. Of course, they said yes. Over the years, I have accumulated thirty-eight recommendations.

I always felt that my clients and candidates would be my most prominent and powerful advocates/cheerleaders. When I speak to a potential new client, I also direct them to the recommendations section of my LinkedIn profile; I sometimes call it my Yelp section. When someone scrolls through the people that have left a recommendation, I usually get the same reaction: "Wow! Very impressive! You have worked with some great people." It makes me think back to my time in LA when I thought, *It's not who you know; it's who knows you!*

I WAS HEADS-DOWN at my desk when Jim stopped in front of my office.

"I need to speak with you. Can you come down to my office in fifteen minutes?" he asked.

"Sure," I said.

Jim turned and walked down the hallway to his office. I sat back in my chair. What did he want to talk about? *I hope it doesn't have anything to do with my recent placements*, I thought with a twinge of anxiety.

Fifteen minutes later, I walked down the hallway to Jim's office and sat down across from him.

Jim leaned back in his chair and folded his hands in his lap. "I wanted to congratulate you again on a great year."

A sigh of relief escaped my lips. "Thank you. For a moment, I thought you were going to tell me something about my placements."

"No!" he said quickly. "Everything is fine. What I wanted to speak to you about is your office. Since you were the top biller last year, you can move back into an office with a window view."

When I'd been performing poorly, I'd been moved into one of the four fishbowl offices. I'd been bummed to lose my office with a view when it happened, but now, as I sat looking at Jim, I thought about my days play-

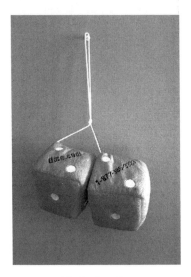

My lucky dice

ing baseball. I am sure you have heard that baseball players are some of the most superstitious people in the world. Well, I was one of those people. In high school, I had to go to McDonald's with my buddy John and have a Filet-O-Fish sandwich with fries and a Coca-Cola before every game I pitched. My good luck charm these days was a pair of fuzzy dice that I'd received from Dice when I was making all those placements at Callidus. I'd pinned the dice on my office door, arranged so you could see the Dice.com name on one of the dice and "snake eyes" below the Dice.com name. I wasn't about to move them and risk disrupting my good luck streak. To this day, I still have that pair of fuzzy dice set up the same way on a wall in my home office.

"Thank you, Jim, but I think I'm going to keep my office," I said.

CHAPTER 86

I'VE ALWAYS BELIEVED IN following your passion when choosing a career. However, I also believe it's essential to recognize that sometimes, despite investing significant time and effort, our initial passion may not materialize as we hoped. In such cases, it becomes crucial to identify areas where we excel and then focus on developing a genuine passion for those pursuits.

When I joined Triad Group in 2001, I was still not 100 percent sure that recruiting was what I should be doing. But now, after experiencing a successful year in recruitment and gaining confidence in my abilities, I consciously decided to embrace my role as a recruiter and channel my passion toward it.

If I wanted to be known as one of the top recruiters, I had to work harder and smarter than everyone else. I was already working hard, of course, but I needed to step it up and do even more to be the best. *It's not the effort, it's the result*, I often reminded myself.

To be a top recruiter in Silicon Valley, I needed to know as much as possible about the top software companies and emerging companies in Silicon Valley, including who the top executives, CEOs, and venture capitalists (VCs) were. To that end, I bought subscriptions to the top business magazines and started spending an hour every morning reading news about software companies in the Bay Area and who was funding startups.

I also decided I needed to be more curious when I had opportunities to speak with tech executives and other brilliant people. (That wouldn't be hard; I had always been naturally curious. Donnita constantly gave me a hard time for always asking her questions that started with "Why . . . ?")

IN THE FIRST three months of 2004, I made five placements at Callidus. The company had gone public in November 2003, and I thought its star would keep rising—but in late March 2004, they announced that it would record a surprise loss in the first quarter due to a shortfall in licensing revenue. At the beginning of 2004, Callidus stock had been trading at $15.78. When the news broke about the company's first-quarter loss, the stock dropped $4.98 (36 percent), plunging to $8.70. Next came the layoffs.

On June 24, Callidus announced that its president and CEO had resigned and an interim president and CEO would be stepping in. It was clear to me after that announcement that Callidus would not be hiring for a while—and if they did, they would be filling the roles with their internal recruiters. I would not make another placement at Callidus anytime soon.

I was a bit worried since I only had two roles to work on at the moment, but I was a wholehearted believer in the idea that as one door closes, another invariably swings wide open. All I could do was keep my eyes open and hope for the best.

CHAPTER 87

June 2004. The phone in my office rang. I picked it up. On the other end was Rob, a product manager from Siebel Software. We'd instantly hit it off the first time we spoke on the phone and started to talk about sports. He'd mentioned that he'd started a sports memorabilia business when he was a little kid and still collected memorabilia, and he'd flipped when I told him I had a baseball signed by the 1973 Oakland A's, a football signed by the 1970s San Francisco 49ers, a signed Joe Montana jersey, and many other autographs by well-known athletes.

Rob and I had spoken a few times the previous year about product marketing roles I was working on, but he hadn't been interested in any of the companies. I kept hoping I could find a role for him. I loved his background. He was in his late twenties and smart. He had a BS from State University of New York at Albany and an MBA from Harvard.

On this call, however, I quickly discovered that I would not be placing Rob anytime soon.

"I called because I wanted to let you know that I recently accepted a role at a startup as the first product marketing hire," he said.

"Congrats!" I said. "What's the name of the company?"

"SuccessFactors."

I had never heard of them, so I started to look them up online.

Rob heard me typing away and quickly said, "Don't look at the website. We are redoing it."

I could see why; the website was horrible. But Rob was a smart guy. If he'd taken a job at this company, there had to be something to it.

"I mentioned your name to the CFO as someone who could help us find great people," Rob said. "He is currently handling recruiting, until we get a director of HR."

"Thank you," I said, touched that he'd thought of me.

"Of course," he said. "Hope something works out."

- - -

A FEW DAYS LATER, I received a call from a person I'd put in front of one of the VPs at Callidus for a role in 2003.

"Well, with their stock looking like it does right now and all the layoffs they're doing, I'm glad now the Callidus opportunity didn't work out for you," I joked.

"Right?" he said, chuckling. "Actually, I just joined a new company as their first product management hire."

"Congrats!" I said. "Which company?"

"SuccessFactors!" he said.

"No way," I said. "Rob Bernshteyn just called me a few days ago, letting me know he was at SuccessFactors."

"Oh yeah, Rob's great," he said.

I had to look into this company. If these two guys were joining SuccessFactors, something interesting must be happening over there.

As soon as we hung up, I started looking into SuccessFactors. I learned that it was founded in 2001 by Aaron Au and Lars Dalgaard and was an on-demand HCM (human capital management) software company. They received $2.13 million in Series A funding in 2003 and $5 million in Series B funding in 2004. Greylock Partners invested in both rounds of funding. They currently did not have an office of their own, so they used space at the Greylock Partners office in San Mateo.

A FEW WEEKS LATER, I spoke with the CFO at SuccessFactors, Steve Bach. He laid out their hiring needs and mentioned that they would be looking for engineers, marketers, and salespeople. I told him I would love to work on any of the open roles.

"We definitely need some help with finding someone for one critical role, Director of Alliances," he said. "We want someone who can build out the whole Alliances function."

As Steve continued describing the type of person they wanted for the role, I wrote a name on my yellow notepad: *Roger Goulart*.

Roger had been VP of Alliances at BroadVision when I was recruiting for them in 2000. He'd left BroadVision in 2002 and gone on to Salesforce, where he became their first VP of Alliances. If anyone knew an up-and-coming Director of Alliances, it was Roger.

The next day I had a signed contract from Steve, and I was off and running on the Director of Alliances search.

I GOT ROGER on the phone as soon as I was able and asked if I could pick his brain. I filled him in on the role and every other pertinent detail I could think of, then asked, "Do you know anyone who might be a fit for this?"

"What is the name of the company?" he asked.

"SuccessFactors."

"Oh."

That caught me off guard. "What do you mean 'oh'? Have you heard of them?"

"I have." He paused. "I do know someone."

I was very excited. This could be a quick placement if Roger gave me a superstar's name. I had my pen and paper ready to write down the name and contact info.

"Who do you have in mind?" I asked.

"Me!" he said.

Now I was thrown even more off guard. "You've been a VP since 1999," I said, totally confused. "This is a director role at a very small startup."

"Do you want to put me in front of them, or should I contact them?" he said.

"Really?"

"Yes, I want to speak to them about the role."

"Okay," I said quickly. "Let me get you in front of them."

On November 1, I placed Roger as VP of Alliances at SuccessFactors. They ended up giving Roger the VP title since he was precisely what they were looking for. I didn't know it yet, but he would be the first of ten people that I would place at SuccessFactors.

THE CEO OF SUCCESSFACTORS, Lars, was always going 110 miles an hour. The first time I met him in the company's new office, he asked me if I wanted something to drink. When I said no thanks, he walked over to the fridge and grabbed a Coca-Cola. "This is my third Coke of the day," he told me as we walked to the conference room. It was 10:00 a.m.

Lars required all new employees at SuccessFactors to sign what he called the "17 rules of engagement." The first time I read the list, I stopped at Rule 14, which read: *I will be a good person to work with—I will not be an asshole.*

I could get behind a rule like that.

Over the next five years, I built relationships with five people at SuccessFactors: Stacey Epstein, Rob Bernshteyn, Steve Bach, Randy Reynolds, and Dave Yarnold. These five people would be instrumental in my success; to this day, they are my biggest cheerleaders.

On November 20, 2007, SuccessFactors had a successful IPO. On December 3, 2011, the company announced that SAP was acquiring them for $3.4 billion.

I'd found my shooting star.

CHAPTER 88

A SECOND DOOR SWUNG OPEN for me in August 2004 when I was contacted by Jon Miller at Epiphany. Located in San Mateo, California, and founded in 1996 as one of the leading developers and vendors of customer relationship management (CRM) software, Epiphany had been one of the many high-flying stocks in the late '90s. The company had gone public in September 1999, and the stock price had soared to $80 a share by the next month. Epiphany stock would rise again to $157.75 a share a month after that. It peaked at $317 a share in early 2000. Unfortunately, by April 2001, the stock had fallen below $10 a share.

Jon was Epiphany's VP of Product Marketing. A VP I had recently worked with had told him I was a good recruiter and could help him with his roles; to start, he wanted my help filling a Senior Director of Solutions Marketing for Financial Services role. We discussed the role and the type of people he thought would be a good fit. He mentioned he would have more roles for me to work on after this one.

After getting off the phone with Jon, I pulled up his profile—and my first reaction was *This is one smart dude!* Jon had an AB in physics from Harvard and an MBA from Stanford and was only in his early thirties.

I'VE LOST COUNT of the number of times I've told Donnita that I never imagined that I would be sitting at a conference table or having dinner with a VP, CEO, or VC who held degrees from the top schools in the world. Interestingly, I've never felt intimidated by those people. I had a breakfast meeting once with a CMO at a crowded restaurant before a big tech conference in San Francisco, and he said, "You seem so relaxed."

Maybe it's my chilled-out California attitude. Maybe it's because I spent so much time around famous athletes and actors in my twenties and thirties. But what I attribute it to is the fact that I was finally at a point in my life where I was not fearful of having a seizure at any moment and having people staring at me as if I were on drugs or a weirdo. During the period of my life when I was having uncontrollable seizures on a regular basis, people would never have told me I seemed relaxed.

I ENDED UP filling all three roles Jon brought to me. For one of the roles, I had the privilege of placing a candidate for the second time in his career. After that happened, I decided to start a club I would call "Double Trouble." Seven years later, I would place a candidate for the third time in their career, and I started a new club called "Triple Threat." I'm looking forward to starting a new club of people that I've placed four times in their career.

The third placement would be the last time I worked with Epiphany, as they were acquired by SSA Global Technologies later in 2005—but it would not be the last time I would work with Jon Miller.

As 2005 ended, some of my coworkers told me I was a great recruiter. I told them I needed ten good years before considering myself a "great" recruiter. I always felt you had to have multiple years of success before you could be regarded as "great" at anything. Many people get lucky and have one or two great years, but the real test is if you can do it year after year after year.

Still, it was exciting to note that I'd had three great years at Triad Group now, with no signs of slowing down. All my hard work in 2002 was finally starting to pay off; I had reached a point where hiring managers were now contacting *me*, rather than the other way around.

My health was excellent as well. I still experienced side effects from the medication (sleepiness and dizziness), but I was scrupulous about taking it every day, and I had developed ways to power through the symptoms.

That winter, after twelve years at The Cheesecake Factory, Donnita decided it was time to move on. She started a teller job at Wells Fargo after the new year. The bank was conveniently located—less than two miles from our house—which played a big part in her decision. She was thrilled to have such an easy commute.

As 2006 started, I started hearing an internal voice conveying a gentle but insistent message: *This is the perfect time to do it.*

CHAPTER 89

STARTING IN 2005, Jim had implemented a President's Club competition for each quarter of the year, the prize for which was a group trip to which you could invite your significant other. The third quarter of 2006 was a huge one, and five of us qualified for the President's Club. Jim discussed a possible destination with everyone who qualified, and we ultimately decided on Las Vegas.

Our group of twelve left for Las Vegas on Tuesday, November 14. The plan was to play golf, see a show, eat at excellent restaurants, and do a little gambling. We stayed at the newly opened The Signature at MGM. The place was beautiful.

Before leaving on our trip, I'd told Jim I would check around and see what shows might be fun. Of course, I was a bit biased. On Wednesday night, we had front-row seats at the Flamingo to see my good friend and favorite comedian, George Wallace. It was a fantastic show.

THE FOLLOWING DAY, during breakfast, Jim informed everyone that he had planned something special for the night.

"Do whatever you want today," he said, "but be in the lobby at five o'clock, ready to go!"

I spent the day playing golf with Jim and two other coworkers. The day flew by, and before I knew it, it was 5:00 p.m.

As we all gathered in the lobby, people started asking Jim what we were doing and where we were going, but he said nothing.

A few minutes after five, a long black stretch Hummer limo slowly pulled up in front of the lobby door. Everybody started looking at each other, clearly wondering, *Is that for us?*

As everyone gazed out the large window, admiring the limo, I approached the large double doors, turned to face the group, and declared, "We're going to a wedding!"

I grabbed Donnita by the hand, and we led the way to the limo, which was filled with ice buckets overflowing with champagne. My bartending instincts kicked in: I popped a bottle of champagne and started filling glasses.

As the limo cruised down South Las Vegas Boulevard, my coworkers inundated me with an avalanche of questions. I grinned mischievously as I unveiled our master plan, divulging that this day had been meticulously plotted for what felt like eons.

It had all begun during a Las Vegas trip we'd made in October, to attend Donnita's friend's wedding. While we were there, I'd told Donnita I wanted to make it official and get married. We'd filled out the marriage license paperwork the day before returning home. Once back in the office, I'd confided in Jim, secretly enlisting him in our plan to have a Las Vegas wedding as part of the President's Club trip. He'd wholeheartedly embraced the notion, vowing to keep our secret as tightly sealed as a blackjack dealer's poker face.

As the champagne flowed and vibrant music emanated from the speakers, our limousine glided gracefully into the parking lot of A Little White Chapel. With a sense of awe and anticipation, Donnita and I contemplated the illustrious history of the iconic venue. It had played host to legendary couples, including Frank Sinatra and Mia Farrow, Demi Moore and Bruce Willis, and Michael Jordan and Juanita Vanoy; surely that made it a fitting setting for our special occasion!

The limo doors swung open.

"Michael, your buddy George is here!" one of my coworkers called out.

I looked out the window and saw George getting out of his Mercedes. "Yep! He will be my best man and our witness."

It was all happening just as we'd planned it.

PEOPLE ALWAYS ASK Donnita and me why we did not have a big wedding.

The truth is, we had only recently gotten out of debt, and we didn't want to spend a lot of money on a wedding. Plus, Donnita had already had the big Cinderella-style wedding on the Queen Mary—and we know how *that* worked out.

Anyway, in our eyes, we'd already been married for years—ever since we'd exchanged rings. This ceremony was to make it legal, and I was delighted to be "officially" married, but we'd already considered ourselves husband and wife for years.

The year 2006 had shaped up to be filled with joyous milestones and remarkable achievements. I married Donnita, continued my success at Triad Group, and continued to live seizure-free. I was grateful every day for my amazing life.

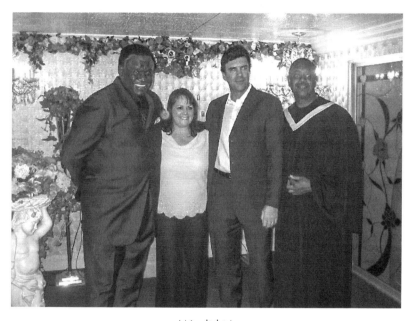

We did it!

CHAPTER 90

DON'T PLAY GOD!

This was one of the many lessons I learned while recruiting for Taleo Software.

Like SuccessFactors, Taleo was in the HCM space, with headquarters east of the San Francisco Bay in Dublin, California. This was my first time working with a company in the East Bay; most software companies at the time were headquartered on the Peninsula, south of San Francisco, in San Francisco proper, or in the South Bay near San Jose.

In early May of 2008, I placed the Senior Director of Marketing, Business Edition at Taleo. That candidate was eventually promoted to VP of Marketing. In 2009, a VP of Product Marketing role opened up at Taleo. I should have been the one to fill it, but I made a critical mistake.

A month into the process, I had five strong candidates in front of the CMO, and he was moving two of my candidates forward to meet a group of executives. If all went well with those interviews, there would be one final interview. I was feeling good about our chances.

Curiosity was driving me crazy, so I reached out to the CMO to see how many other candidates he had in front of the group of executives.

"I have your two candidates this far along in the process," he told me.

Score! I thought.

My good feeling quickly changed, however, when he said, "But I have another candidate that looks good that applied online yesterday. I am going to try to put him through the process quickly. I believe you may know him."

"Really?" I asked. "Who is it?"

My jaw dropped when he said the name. I had known this person since 2003; in fact, he was a superstar.

I looked down at my list of potential candidates for the Taleo role. There was his name—but it was crossed out. Next to his name, I'd written, *Burlingame is too far. He's too senior for the role.*

I hadn't even contacted him about the role because (1) I'd assumed he would never want to make that commute, and (2) he had been a CEO and VP over the last seven years; this role didn't feel big enough for him.

In August 2009, he was hired as Taleo's VP of Product Marketing.

A few months later, I was in town and invited him to meet me for breakfast at the Sofitel Hotel in Redwood City.

The first thing I said when he arrived was "Congrats on the role at Taleo."

"Thank you," he said. "You should have called me about that role!"

"I know, I know," I said, shaking my head. "I learned my lesson."

After that meeting, I decided it was not my place to decide how far someone was willing to commute or whether they'd think they were too senior for the role I was working on. That's when I coined the phrase *Don't play God!*

IN 2013, SINCE I was no longer "playing God," I contacted a candidate about a Senior Director of Product Marketing role at DocuSign. The candidate was very senior; he'd nabbed his first director role in 1999 and had landed a VP of Marketing role in 2006. But DocuSign was a fast-growing, pre-IPO company, and the role reported to the VP of Product Marketing, who I personally knew to be a terrific guy.

After meeting my candidate for the first time, the VP of Product Marketing agreed that he was the perfect person for the role. My candidate joined DocuSign as the Senior Director of Product Marketing and was eventually promoted to VP of Product Marketing.

Over the years, I have spoken to many people about roles that were technically either a lateral move or even a step down from their current title. But as I always tell people, "It's not the title going in; it's the title coming out!" My placement at DocuSign was the perfect example of that.

CHAPTER 91

On Monday, September 15, 2008, at 1:45 a.m., Lehman Brothers filed for Chapter 11 bankruptcy protection, triggering a catastrophic ripple effect. The Dow plummeted 504 points, which would be the equivalent of a staggering 1,300 points today. The aftermath saw a whopping $700 billion vanish from retirement plans and investment funds, sending shockwaves through the economy and culminating in what is now recognized as the Great Recession.

Throughout the first half of 2008, there was a glimmer of hope that the tech sector could withstand the recessionary pressures; I had three big quarters in a row and once again made President's Club. But as 2008 ended and the economy continued its downward trend domestically and internationally, consumer and corporations' demand for technology products and services sharply declined, and tech firms had to lay people off.

Unfortunately, the outlook for 2009 seemed equally grim. Analysts foresaw a potential escalation in layoffs throughout the year, citing a lack of evidence to suggest that the economy had hit the bottom of this downward cycle.

During the first three months of 2009, the tech sector suffered the deepest layoffs it had seen in seven years. Once again, I encountered that familiar old refrain from hiring managers, echoing the sentiments I had heard back in 2001 and 2002: "Sorry, Michael, I can't engage outside agencies at the moment."

As the first quarter ended and a company-wide email from Jim arrived, notifying us about a meeting to be held at 9:00 a.m. on Friday morning, April 3, I couldn't stop thinking about the company-wide meeting we'd had at Littler Savage during the last big tech downturn. It was difficult to focus on anything else for the remainder of the day.

As I drove into work on April 3, my mind was filled with thoughts about the topics Jim might discuss during our meeting. I'd barely slept the previous night, and my thoughts were really running wild. Was he going to lay people off? Was he going to shut down the company?

I was way down the rabbit hole by the time I pulled into the parking lot and made my way to our floor.

Once in my office, I quickly checked my emails before heading into the conference room for our meeting. There were more than forty messages in my inbox, but unfortunately none were from hiring managers. They were all from people who had been laid off and were looking for jobs.

Discouraged, I left my office and walked into the conference room.

As I entered the conference room, I could feel the negative energy. Everyone in the company had had a bad Q1, and none of us had much hope of things improving anytime soon.

Jim entered the room and sat down at the head of the table. I scrutinized his face but couldn't tell if he was about to give us good or bad news.

"Morning!" he said.

"Morning!" we replied in unison.

"I wanted to call this meeting because there have been rumors running around the office that I'm going to have to let go of some people who are not performing," he said, "as well as rumors that I'm going to shut down the company." He looked around the table, meeting our gazes. "This is not my first downturn. Just like the previous downturns I've experienced, things will come back; they always have. I want to assure everyone that I will not be letting go of anyone, and I'm certainly not shutting down the company."

A smile slowly appeared on my face, and as I surveyed the table, I saw my fellow recruiters relax their previously tense bodies—shoulders dropped, foreheads softened.

Jim rose from his chair. "This meeting is over. That's all I wanted to discuss. Let's get back to work." He exited the conference room.

After Jim left, I sat there for a few minutes with my coworkers, discussing other possible ways the meeting could have gone. We were all glad that we still had jobs.

CHAPTER 92

WHEN IS A GOOD TIME to start a company or be a first-time CEO? The answer is now! There is no such thing as waiting for the "right time."

With everything that was happening in 2009—foreclosures on the rise, the unemployment rate at 10 percent, banks closing, and the S&P 500 below 700—you would think it wouldn't have been the best time to start a company or take your first CEO role.

But maybe it was the perfect time.

In 2009, many new companies decided there was no time like the present to start their business. These included WhatsApp, Groupon, Slack, Uber, Square, and Okta.

Also in 2009, two people I had previously worked with decided to jump at the opportunity to become a first-time CEO—including Rob Bernshteyn.

In February 2009, Rob became the CEO of Coupa, an on-demand spend management startup founded in 2006 by two Oracle alumni, Dave Stephens and Noah Eisner. When Rob joined, there were only nineteen employees, and the company's revenue from the previous year was a few hundred thousand dollars.

During this time, I noticed that companies with "nice to have" products were struggling, and those with "must have" products, like security software, were still flourishing. Products that helped companies save money or track spending were also doing quite well. Coupa's mission was simple: empowering organizations to spend smarter and save money. Their cloud-based spend management applications were easy to use, fast to implement, and cost-effective,

Maybe this was the perfect time to be the CEO at Coupa.

Coupa received $1.5 million in their Series A in 2007 and $6 million in their Series B in 2008. In September 2009, Rob helped Coupa secure $7.5 million in Series C funding.

In 2011, Rob contacted me to help him find his VP of Marketing. After working with many startups, I'd realized the main reason someone should or should not join a startup wasn't the VCs who funded the company, the product, or the space the company was in—it was the person running the show, the CEO. So, when I spoke to candidates about Coupa, I asked them, "If you went to the horse races and were going to bet on a race, would you bet on the jockey or the horse?" I told the candidates that this opportunity was about betting on the jockey, and his name was Rob Bernshteyn.

During the search, all the candidates would ask me the same question: "What is Rob's exit strategy? Does he want to get acquired, or does he want to have an IPO?"

Rob and I had discussed this before I started the search because I knew people would ask me this question. I loved Rob's answer: "I want to build the best company I can build, and then we will see what happens once I've done that." This seemed to satisfy most candidates.

I presented several strong candidates for the role, and one of them stood out to Rob. He asked me to set up a phone call with her. After he spoke with her on the phone, he sent me an email letting me know he'd enjoyed the conversation and wanted to have her come in and meet a few people.

When I called the candidate to get her availability to meet more people at Coupa, her lukewarm response surprised me.

"Yeah, I don't think I'm interested in the opportunity," she told me. "Rob seems like a great guy, but I'm just not excited about the spend management space."

I tried to convince her to at least go into the office and meet more people. I kept telling her that the reason to join Coupa was Rob's vision and drive to succeed. She didn't agree and decided to stay at her current company. (For the record—I spoke to her a few years ago, and she brought up Coupa's success and said, "I should have listened to you.")

So, unfortunately, I didn't place the VP of Marketing at Coupa. But after the new VP of Marketing was hired, Rob did ask me to help him build his marketing team, which I gladly did.

Rob would raise another $154 million in funding at Coupa over the years. In 2016, Coupa's revenue would grow to $84 million, and it would have a successful IPO in October of that year.

On the day of Coupa's IPO, I invested $25,000. In February 2021, when Coupa stock hit $350 a share, I sold it all.

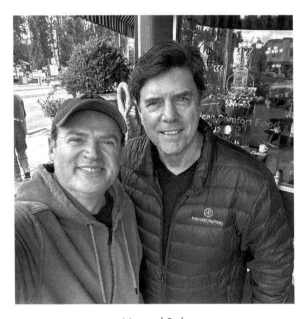

Me and Rob

CHAPTER 93

I WAS INTRODUCED to Dave Yarnold back in 2005 by Steve Bach, the CFO at SuccessFactors. Steve sent an email introducing us and letting Dave know that I could help him find some strong account executives to add to his team. When I saw the name Dave Yarnold, it rang a bell—and not one from my professional life.

Before responding to the email, I called my childhood friend Chris.

"Do you know what Dave Yarnold is doing these days?" I asked him.

"The last I heard about Dave, he was in sales at some tech company."

Bam! This was the Dave Yarnold from junior high!

Dave and I weren't close friends in school, but we certainly knew each other. When he and I spoke on the phone a couple of days later, we had a great conversation reminiscing about the Ben Franklin Junior High and Westmoor High School days and catching up on what he had been doing and what I had been doing since then.

In April 2009, Dave decided to take the plunge as a first-time CEO and joined Maxplore Technologies (later rebranded to ServiceMax), a startup that provided field service management software for equipment manufacturers and service providers. They received their Series A funding, a $2 million round led by Emergence Capital, in 2008. When Dave joined, the ARR was less than $1 million, with five employees and twenty customers. A year later, Dave secured a Series B round of funding for $8 million.

One of the first people Dave hired was Stacey Epstein. Stacey had first worked for Dave in 1997 when he'd been the VP of Sales at Clarify, and they'd worked together again when Stacey joined SuccessFactors as the Senior Director of Marketing Communications role in 2005.

In December 2014, Stacey called to inform me that she was leaving ServiceMax to join a small social media startup as their CMO. After chatting with her about her decision for a while, I decided it was time to put on my recruiter hat.

"Has Dave retained someone to find your replacement?" I asked.

"Not yet," she said. "But I told Dave he should have you work on finding my replacement. You should reach out to him."

"Thank you for thinking of me," I said. "I'll reach out to him."

Dave and I spoke on the phone a week later, and he retained me to find his next CMO.

"How well do you know the CEO at ServiceMax?"

I always heard that question during my conversations with potential CMO candidates, and I don't blame them; I would have done the same thing. When asked that question, I always wished I was on a video call with the person so I could see their reaction to my answer. Since it was a phone call, I only got an awkward silence when I answered, "I have known Dave since seventh grade."

I'm sure their awkward silence was them thinking, *He didn't really say SEVENTH GRADE, did he?*

Of course, I had a lot of interesting conversations with people from there.

When Dave and I first spoke about the type of person he was looking for in his CMO, he was very specific. Since they were on pace for an IPO, he wanted someone who had taken a company public. He also wanted someone who had worked at a SaaS (software as a service) company and had taken a company to over $100 million in ARR, and he wanted them to be in the office every day.

I was glad to hear that Dave knew exactly the type of background he wanted in his CMO. I constantly get asked why the tenure for CMOs and VPs of Marketing is so short, and my answer is always the same: "The CEO has no clue about what kind of background is needed for where the company's at right now."

Companies are at different stages of growth and revenue, so you need to hire a CMO or VP of Marketing that fits your stage. Too many times, I have seen CEOs at Series A or Series B companies hire someone from a big-brand tech company and think they made a great hire. Wrong! What does that person know about scaling revenue from $0 to $10 million or from $20 million to $30 million? When I work on CMO or VP of Marketing searches for Series A or Series B companies, I tell the CEO, "I'm going to get you someone that has played in and excelled in the 'startup sandbox.' If they have never played in the sandbox, I will not put them in front of you."

It was time to go CMO hunting!

Like all my searches for companies in the East Bay, I first focused on people who lived there and had taken a company public. That list was pretty short. Next, I made a list of everyone I could think of who had taken a company public, period, regardless of where they lived in the Bay Area. I emailed those people on my list and then went on LinkedIn to see if I could find more good candidates.

After lots of calls and consideration, I put three candidates in front of Dave. A few weeks later, one of the people I'd emailed who lived in the East Bay and had taken a company public before got back to me. Over his career, he had been a CMO at large-enterprise software companies and fast-growing startups. He'd taken his current company public in 2014. He was open to discussing the role at ServiceMax since his current company stock price had recently sunk to under $4 a share.

He was perfect for the role. I presented him to Dave right away, and Dave loved him.

Then the hammer fell: my candidate let me know that although he was excited about the opportunity at ServiceMax, he felt sure his current company stock price was going to double by the end of the year, and he thought that it would be a mistake to leave now. I tried everything to convince him that ServiceMax was on track to have an IPO by the end of 2016 or sooner, but he stood his ground—he was pulling himself out of the interview process and staying at his current company.

Like that, I was back to square one.

OVER THE FOLLOWING MONTHS I put candidate after candidate in front of Dave, but he found each one lacking. None were as strong as the candidate who'd pulled out of the interview process. He had definitely set the bar high.

Eventually, Dave let me know that he'd decided to have another firm help with the search. "I figure having two places look for me increases my chances of finding the right person," he said bluntly. He also decided to bring on a consultant to help hold down the fort until he found his CMO.

I understood his reasoning, but I was frustrated that I could not find the perfect candidate for him.

I HAD MADE PLANS earlier in the year to be in the Bay Area from September 13 through September 20 to meet with companies, candidates, family, and friends. I decided to email the candidate who'd pulled out of the interview process and ask if he was open to meeting me in San Francisco.

He got back to me and said he could meet me for breakfast at The Ritz-Carlton on Tuesday the fifteenth. Perfect.

I wanted to meet with him because I'd been keeping track, and I knew his company's stock had not doubled as he had thought it would. The stock price had increased by two dollar a share for a while but was now back below four. I hoped I could convince him to reengage in the CMO search at ServiceMax.

I ARRIVED AT THE RITZ-CARLTON right at 9:00 a.m. on September 15 for our breakfast. After we'd gone through all the usual pleasantries, he jumped right in: "How's the CMO search going at ServiceMax?"

"It's moving along," I said. "I have put some great people in front of Dave, but he has not pulled the trigger on anyone just yet. He decided to hire a consultant to keep things moving, and he's trying to convince them to join full time."

This last part wasn't true; Dave had actually said the person was not looking for a full-time role. But I decided to keep that information to myself.

"I noticed that the stock price at your company went up a bit for a while, but now it's right back to under four dollars a share," I said.

He took a sip of his coffee and didn't say anything.

Guess he doesn't want to talk about that! I took a bite of my huevos rancheros and thought about how to proceed. After a pause, I said, "Let me ask you a question. When you are getting ready in the morning to go to work and look in the mirror as you brush your teeth, shave, and comb your hair, are you looking forward to going to work?"

He chuckled. "You sound like my wife."

I got a kick out of his response, but I wasn't going to let him get away with not answering. "Well, what's your answer?"

He took another sip of his coffee and finally said, "No. I am not excited to go to work."

Perfect! That was exactly the response I had been anticipating. Though inwardly elated, I masked my emotions and simply said in a composed tone, "Life is too short not to be excited about where you work."

Fork in hand, he moved his eggs from side to side on his plate. I could tell that he had been thinking about that too.

"Let me ask you another question," I proposed. "Would you be open to having another conversation with Dave?"

He looked down at his empty mug and motioned to the server for more coffee. After his cup had been refreshed, he added sugar and cream and circled the inside of his cup with his spoon slowly. Finally, he nodded. "Yes, I would like to speak to Dave again about the CMO role at ServiceMax."

On October 28, he signed his offer to become the new CMO at ServiceMax.

That placement broke the Triad Group company record for the largest permanent placement in the company's history, breaking the previous record—which I set in December 2014 when I placed the VP of Global Devops Marketing at CA Technologies. It seemed I'd really found my groove.

IN 2017, WHEN I WAS IN the Bay Area to meet with candidates I had placed, I met up with Dave Yarnold in San Francisco to catch up—and to celebrate ServiceMax's recent acquisition for almost $1 billion.

I met Dave at the W Hotel on 3rd Street across from Moscone Center. I found him in the back right corner, already sipping on a cocktail.

We greeted each other with a big hug and sat down.

"What are you drinking?" I asked.

Dave held up his glass. "Rye old-fashioned."

Our server spotted me and made her way over to our table. "What can I get you to drink?" she asked.

"A negroni, please."

When my drink arrived, I raised my glass and said, "Congrats! Not bad for a boy from DC."

"Thank you!" Dave smiled. "Not bad for *two* boys from DC. Congrats on all of your success, Michael."

We touched glasses. As I sipped my drink, I thought of all the people I had met and placed over the years who were once senior managers or directors and are now VPs and CEOs. One day, I decided to start a new club called "I Knew You When." Of course, number one on the list was Dave Yarnold.

Looking at Dave, I couldn't help but think back to seventh grade at Ben Franklin Junior High. Back then, I never would have thought I would be sitting at a bar in San Francisco with Dave Yarnold, celebrating our success, almost forty-five years later.

You never know who will come in and out of your life.

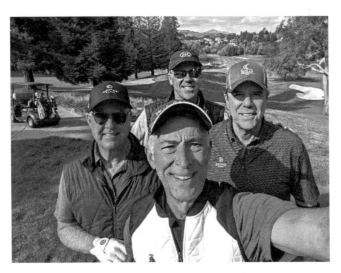

DC Boys – Jay, Chris, Dave and Me

CHAPTER 94

IT WAS A RAINY SEATTLE DAY in 2009, and I knew traffic into work would be horrible, so I quickly gobbled the last scoops of my Honey Nut Cheerios with sliced bananas, grabbed my glass of OJ, and walked over to a kitchen cabinet. It was time to take my medication—the same medication I had been taking religiously since my surgery in 1998.

I reached up, took the pill bottle from the shelf, placed two pills in the palm of my right hand, and looked down at them. I had been seizure-free for eleven years. The side effects of Tegretol—drowsiness, dizziness, and overall lack of energy—had been part of my existence since I started taking the medication in 1992. I looked down at the two pills one more time. Then I lifted my right hand and slowly slid one of the pills back into the bottle. I popped the other pill into my mouth, washed it down with the OJ, and left for work.

IN 1998, MY DOCTORS at UCLA had told me I would need to take medicine for the rest of my life—that if I didn't stick to the plan, I might have more seizures. I'd had many conversations with myself over the years about whether I should mess with my medication or not. Now that I was doing it, I was thrilled not to feel any signs that I might have a seizure.

Over the next four months, I gradually weaned myself off my medication one pill at a time. As time passed, I started feeling more energetic. Feeling confident, I decided to stay off my medicine for good, as long as my seizures remained at bay. I also decided not to tell my doctor or Donnita I had stopped taking my medication. This would be my own private victory over my health journey.

DISCLAIMER: I WOULD *never advocate for anyone who is taking medication to control their seizures to wean themselves off their medication or to stop taking their medication. I did this on my own, knowing that it was a risky choice. I do not support anyone else trying this.*

CHAPTER 95

Is there a perfect time to buy a house?

When the housing market crashed in 2009, I thought that maybe now was the perfect time to move back to the Bay Area and buy a house. All of my business was in the Bay Area, and I'd long wondered if I would make more money if I lived there. I could meet people for coffee and lunch and even play golf with potential clients and candidates. I might even make unexpected connections if, say, I were coaching Natalie's softball or basketball team and some of the other parents happened to be executives at software companies.

It was May 2009, and although the hiring market was slowing down, I flew to San Francisco to meet with clients and candidates and, of course, see my family and friends. I had a great trip—and it made me wonder about moving even more.

When I arrived back in Seattle, Donnita was there waiting to pick me up in the pouring rain—a stark contrast to the perfect weather I'd experienced in the Bay.

It continued to be cloudy and rainy for the next three weeks. The weather was really starting to get to me.

One night at dinner, I looked at Donnita and said, "I want to move back to the Bay Area."

When we'd moved to Seattle in 2001, Donnita had told me, "If you are ever not happy here, we can move."

It was official: I was not happy.

Over the next few weeks, we discussed the different cities in the Bay Area where we might want to move—Concord, Walnut Creek, Clayton, and Lafayette.

Donnita loved where we lived and had thought we would never move, but she was true to her promise: she went along with me, looking on Redfin for homes in those areas.

Home prices in the Bay Area had gone down during the economic dip, but they were still much higher than they were in the Issaquah area. We had been able to pay off all our debt in 2006 by rotating our credit card debt into balance transfers at 0 percent interest. We both had excellent credit, and I'd been able to put some money aside over the last few years. Since the recruiting business had slowed down, maybe now wasn't the best time to buy a house—but maybe it was.

We sat at our dining room table one night, and I pulled out two pieces of paper. At the top of one of the pieces of paper, I wrote *Bay Area*. I then drew a line down the middle of the paper. On the left side, I wrote *Positive*. On the right side, I wrote *Negative*. On the second piece of paper, I wrote *Issaquah* and again divided it into positive and negative sides.

I started by listing the positive reasons for moving to the Bay Area.

For me, the positives were sunshine, family, friends, and business. The business part was, of course, the big "if." Would I make more money if I lived in the Bay Area? If so, how much more money would I need to make to have it all make sense? Those were the two million-dollar questions.

Now for the negatives: state income tax, higher cost of living, smaller house compared to Issaquah, public schools not as good as Issaquah schools, and more traffic.

I switched to the Issaquah paper and listed the positives: can buy a bigger house, no state income tax, great schools, Donnita's family. For negatives, I only wrote one word, in all caps: *WEATHER*.

Donnita looked over the lists on both sides of the paper and circled *sunshine* on the Bay Area paper and *WEATHER* on the Issaquah paper.

"It seems like the big thing for you is sunshine," she said.

"It is." I nodded vigorously. "One of the reasons I wanted to move to LA in the first place was the weather. I was done with all the fog."

Donnita started doodling on the Issaquah paper. "I have an idea. Why don't we look at bigger homes in the Issaquah area, and you and I can get sunshine when we want it?"

After talking it over for a few days, we decided to stay in Issaquah and look for a bigger house. It just made sense to stay there, where I could make money off the outrageous Bay Area salaries without having the overhead of living in the Bay Area. We agreed that I could make more business trips to the Bay Area to get sunshine, and we could travel to sunny places like Arizona and Palm Springs more often with the money we would save by staying in Issaquah.

It wasn't perfect, but it felt like a pretty good solution, all told.

CHAPTER 96

WE WERE MORE OPPORTUNISTIC home buyers than serious buyers. We loved our house in Issaquah, but if we could find a "too good to pass up" home, we would pull the trigger.

I started looking on Redfin for homes in Issaquah and found nothing I liked or that looked like a great deal. Eventually, I got to a point where the idea of buying a bigger house when the prices were dropping was starting to feel like a dream.

Then, one day, I pulled up Redfin to see if there were any new listings while I was eating lunch at work—and bam! There was a house for sale in one of the prized neighborhoods only five minutes from our house.

SE Issaquah–Fall City Road is a thirteen-mile road that starts at East Lake Sammamish Parkway SE and makes its way up the hill—or "the plateau," as the locals call it. As you make your way up the hill, there are different neighborhoods, and much like in other places, the neighborhoods get more expensive as you go higher up the plateau. Our neighborhood was located about halfway up the plateau. The house on Redfin was nestled in a neighborhood right at the top, with unbelievable views of the Cascade Mountains.

We were familiar with the area since Natalie attended the neighborhood's elementary school, and we knew some people who lived there. I would describe the neighborhood as a gated community without a gate—there was one way in and one way out. We'd always dreamed of living in that neighborhood but knew we could never afford it. During the height of the housing market boom, the homes were selling from $800,00 to over $1 million. But now, as I looked at the house for sale on Redfin, I had to blink my eyes twice. I couldn't believe what I was reading; the house was for sale for $621,000.

I looked up the address. It was on a cul-de-sac, less than a mile from Natalie's school. I grabbed the phone and called Donnita.

"Hello?"

"I just found a house for sale on Redfin," I blurted. I told her the neighborhood and that the house was in a cul-de-sac and close to Natalie's school.

"We can't afford a house in that neighborhood," Donnita said.

"It's only $621,000!" I said.

"That can't be right."

But it was; there was the number, in black and white. And once I convinced Donnita, she was as excited as I was. "Let's go see it this weekend!" she suggested.

"Definitely," I agreed.

WE WENT TO the open house on Saturday before Natalie's soccer game. The house was in pristine condition, with a freshly painted interior, hardwood floors, and beautiful Italian stone on the floor of the master bathroom.

Of course, I had to ask the agent the question on both our minds: "Why are they selling?"

"They had no plans to move, but the husband got a promotion at his job that requires him to move to the East Coast," she said with a shrug. "So they're selling."

It was almost too good to be true. It had everything we would ever want in a home—3,100 square feet, three bedrooms, three baths, a media room, an office, and a huge backyard. The house sat on a quarter of an acre. This was our opportunity to move into the neighborhood we'd long loved but never thought we could afford.

We knew a realtor who would do the paperwork for 1 percent of the deal. We called him, and he put together everything we needed to make an offer on the house—$621,000. We put in $12,000 as an earnest money deposit with the offer and started hoping.

A FEW DAYS later, our realtor called and told us we'd gotten the house for $621,000. We were pre-approved for a thirty-year mortgage. Now, we "just" had to pull together $111,000 for the down payment.

We first took out a HELOC (Home Equity Line of Credit) on our house for $50,000. After we'd also taken $41,000 out of our savings (which was scary, because it stretched us out), we were still short $20,000—and we weren't sure how we were going to get it. My parents and Donnita's parents were not in a place where they could loan us the money.

There was only one other person I could think of whom I could ask.

CHAPTER 97

I SAT AT MY DESK in my office and tried to figure out other ways to get the $20,000. I really wanted to buy this house, but maybe it was just not meant to be. Maybe we were stretching ourselves out too much. What would happen if the remainder of 2009 was just as bad as the first part? What would happen if the slowdown continued into 2010?

One of my coworkers popped into my office. "So . . . did you get the house?" he asked.

"I'm working on it," I said. "Getting close."

I sat at my desk for a few more minutes before standing up and walking down the hallway to Jim's office. He was on the phone, but he waved me in. I shut the door behind me, sat down, and waited for him to finish his call.

As soon as he got off the phone, he asked, "Did you get the house?"

"Yes, we did!" I said.

"Congratulations!" he said.

I braced myself. "I need a favor."

He leaned back in his chair. "What do you need?"

"We are twenty thousand dollars short on the down payment." I took a long, deep breath, then let it out in a puff. "I was wondering if there is any way you could loan us twenty thousand dollars, and I will pay it back to you in a year."

I did it. I asked him. Over the last few days, I'd practiced a hundred different ways to make this ask. Now it was done.

Jim did not hesitate. "I can arrange that for you."

All the weight I'd been carrying lifted right off my shoulders. "You have no idea how much this means to me," I said, extending my hand in heartfelt gratitude. "Thank you, thank you!"

"Happy to help," Jim said.

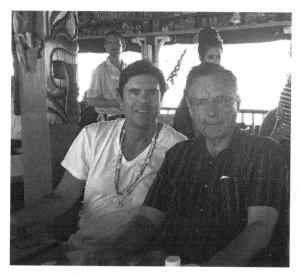

Me and Jim – President Club – Maui - 2014

WE MOVED INTO our new house on June 1. We were still not 100 percent sure what we wanted to do with our house. The price had dropped back down to what we'd paid for it in 2003—$314,000. Should we sell it, or should we try to rent it? One of my coworkers had a rental property and always complained about his tenants. I was not sure I wanted to be a landlord.

We couldn't just let it sit, though, so we decided to go ahead and try renting. The same day we moved into the new house, an ex-teacher who was tutoring Natalie signed a lease and moved into our house. She turned out to be a fantastic tenant, and we never regretted the decision.

As October of 2009 ended, I had not made a placement since April. My clients were still not hiring, and if companies did have an open role, they didn't want to pay me a fee to find that person. I lay in bed many nights, staring at the ceiling, wondering if things would ever pick up again. What worried me the most was that we'd just used almost all of our savings to buy our new house.

Have we made a huge mistake?

CHAPTER 98

Two weeks later, I received an exciting email:

Michael – Are you going to be in town for Dreamforce? I have five marketing roles that I am going to open up. I want to discuss the roles with you.

I replied immediately:

Yes! I will be in town for Dreamforce. Let me know when you want to meet.

Dreamforce is the annual tech conference in San Francisco put on by Salesforce. Salesforce held its first Dreamforce conference in 2003 at the Westin St. Francis Hotel in San Francisco. Over a thousand people showed up to that one. In 2005, the conference expanded and moved over to Moscone Center. One of the main reasons for the move to Moscone Center was that the CEO and co-founder of Salesforce, Mark Benioff, wanted Dreamforce to be the largest attended tech conference, so he issued a large number of free passes. The pass would get you into the expo hall and the kickoff keynote with Marc and his keynote speaker guests. Attendance skyrocketed over the years. After 135,000 people showed up in 2014, Salesforce partnered with Celebrity Cruises and had a cruise ship docked at Pier 27 for Dreamforce 2015—over 150,000 people attended. Marc Benioff got his wish as Dreamforce became the largest technology conference in the world.

Salesforce always attracted fantastic speakers, top entertainers, and bands. Over all these years, the speaker who impacted me most significantly was Microsoft's new CEO, Satya Nadella. At Dreamforce 2015, Satya would be the first person from Microsoft to ever appear at Dreamforce. During this time, Microsoft was having problems. Windows 8 had been a disaster, and consumers and developers were losing faith in the company.

As I sat in the audience, Marc Benioff announced Satya's name to the capacity crowd. Satya walked onto the stage wearing jeans, a black crew neck T-shirt, and a fitted black blazer while rocking the coolest pair of brown patent leather low-top sneakers. As he walked across the stage, I thought, *He doesn't look like a Microsoft CEO.* The image I've always had of a Microsoft CEO was from the famous 1995 Microsoft Windows 95 launch party video where Steve Ballmer (CEO) and Bill Gates showed off their dance moves.

When the keynote speaker session was over, I walked outside to check my emails. I then called Donnita. When she picked up, I said, "You know that twenty thousand dollars we were looking to invest?"

"Yes."

"I want to buy Microsoft. I just listened to the new CEO."

"Okay."

After I hung up, I bought $20,000 worth of Microsoft stock, which I still own to this day.

AT DREAMFORCE 2009, the guest speaker was Colin Powell. After listening to his keynote speech, I went to the expo hall to meet with the hiring manager who wanted my help hiring five marketers for his team. As I entered, I had to dodge the hoard of people who had signed up for the free Expo pass to grab the "swag" companies were giving away at their booths. As I watched the frenzy, I thought, *I'm sure all that stuff will be for sale tonight on eBay.*

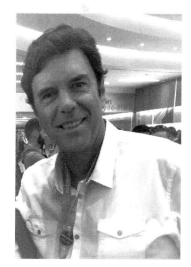

Dreamforce 2009

I finally made my way down a small, crowded aisle with booths of small startups positioned next to each other. I saw my guy standing in front of the booth with a few coworkers. The name on the top of the booth read MARKETO.

It was Jon Miller, who I had worked with in 2004 when he was at Epiphany. In January 2006, Jon and two ex-Epiphany executives (Phil Fernandez and David

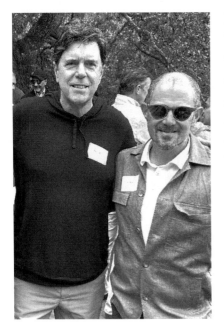

Me and Jon

Morandi) had founded Marketo. The vision was to help CMOs and their teams demonstrate the return on investment from their marketing programs. Marketo had received $10 million in funding for its Series C in September, and Jon was ready to build out his team.

I hung out at the booth with Jon for a while, then we walked to a table and sat down to discuss the roles he wanted help with. John opened his laptop and showed me a spreadsheet of his current team, then showed me the roles he wanted me to fill. We went over them one by one, in detail. I had placed similar roles numerous times, so I knew I had all the ammo I needed to find Jon what he was looking for.

"I've got this," I assured him. "I'll find you some great people."

I RETURNED TO my office after my trip to the Bay Area, feeling exhausted and accomplished. Jim walked into my office.

"How was your trip?" he inquired, leaning casually against the doorframe.

"Busy, but productive. I had some great meetings. I have a full plate of roles now, with more coming next quarter," I replied, mustering a smile despite my fatigue.

"Good to hear."

Before I'd left for my trip, I noticed Nick, one of our recruiters, had not been around. His continued absence sparked a curiosity.

I finally broached the subject, unable to ignore the concern gnawing at me. "Hey, Jim, what's going on with Nick? He's been out for quite a while."

Jim closed the door behind him and took a seat, his expression somber.

"Nick's wife was diagnosed with epilepsy while you were away. He's taking time off to be with her," Jim explained softly, his voice filled with empathy.

The news hit me like a wave, stirring up memories I had long kept buried. It was time to share my own story.

"Jim, I haven't shared this with anyone here, but I've been through something similar. I was diagnosed with epilepsy in 1992 and had surgery in 1997. I've been seizure-free since the surgery," I confessed, the admission feeling both relieving and daunting.

Jim's eyes widened in surprise, but his gaze softened with understanding.

"Would you be comfortable talking to Nick about it? I think it could really help him," Jim asked, his concern evident.

"Yes, absolutely. I'll reach out to him, share my experience, and let him know I'm here if he or his wife needs anything," I replied, a newfound sense of purpose stirring within me.

"Thank you," Jim said sincerely, rising from his chair to leave.

Later that day, I reached out to Nick, sharing my story and offering a listening ear. And as I made the decision to open up to some of my coworkers, I realized that sometimes it's in our vulnerabilities that we find our greatest strengths and connections.

As 2009 ENDED, it hurt to know that I'd only placed four people in the entire year. I was used to placing at least four people in a quarter—and by this point our emergency savings had shrunk to an amount that made me nervous. I needed 2010 to be a big year for my family and me.

CHAPTER 99

It had been eight months since I'd first started weaning myself off my medication. It was a beautiful summer day, and the weather was heating up. Donnita wanted to visit her parents in East Wenatchee for a long weekend. She said I could play golf with her dad, go out on her dad's boat, and do some fishing. I was all in for the golf and the boating; the fishing was for Natalie, Donnita, and her dad.

"Do you mind driving?" Donnita asked.

I was a little surprised, since she usually liked to drive. And in the back of my mind, I was thinking about the fact that I wasn't taking my medication anymore. But Donnita didn't know that. "Sure," I said. "Happy to. Which way do you want to go?"

We had two route options: the wide-open highway I-90 or the more picturesque US 2, which winds through the Cascade Mountains and Stevens Pass.

"Let's take 2!" Donnita said.

We packed the car and began our two-and-a-half-hour journey to East Wenatchee.

After driving for over an hour and a half, we ascended the Cascade Mountains toward Stevens Pass. The road twisted and turned sharply, hugging the contours of the mountainside. The path was narrow, with guardrails protecting us from steep drop-offs. The elevation gain was noticeable, and we climbed higher and higher with each twist.

I took my time as we made our way over the pass. *I better not have a seizure*, I kept thinking.

Forty-five minutes later, we arrived at Donnita's parents' house, and I breathed a sigh of relief.

We had a great weekend with Donnita's parents. I played a great round of golf—I broke 80—and we spent the rest of the day on the lake. Even though East Wenatchee is only 140 miles from Issaquah, the weather is drastically different. Since it was a hundred degrees, time on the water was very much needed. I mainly swam while Natalie, Donnita, and Gerry fished. Donnita and Natalie both caught two fish, which Donnita's dad prepared for dinner, along with the fish he caught.

All in all, a great weekend.

As the sun set on Sunday, we loaded the car up to drive back to Sammamish. Within thirty minutes of being on the road, Donnita and Natalie were asleep. As I drove over the winding Stevens Pass, I couldn't help but tighten my grip on the steering wheel. Just because I hadn't had a seizure in twelve years didn't mean I wouldn't have one now. *After all*, I thought, *I lived for thirty-one years before I had my first one.* Would I even be aware of it if I did have one?

I made it through the pass, and the rest of the drive home was smooth sailing.

I was amazed by the surge I'd experienced in my energy levels since getting off my medication. As I made the long drive home, a trip that would have been challenging on Tegretol, my conviction grew stronger. I firmly concluded that I was healed, dispelling any fears of having another seizure, and I wholeheartedly committed to staying off my medication.

As I pulled into the driveway, I kept looking at Donnita, still sleeping peacefully.

Should I tell her I weaned myself off my medication?

I decided to keep my little secret to myself.

CHAPTER 100

TWO WEEKS LATER, Donnita had my glass of red wine waiting for me on the kitchen table when I got home from work. After I hugged and kissed her, I went upstairs to change into sweatpants and a T-shirt, then came back and sat at the table to enjoy my glass of wine.

As Donnita stirred the food in the pan before her with a wooden spoon, she said, "I noticed that you were getting low on your medication, so I called it in for you."

I took a deep breath, exhaled slowly, and took a sip of wine. I didn't answer her.

She turned toward me. "Did you hear me?"

I didn't know what to say. Should I just say "thank you" and continue to keep my secret? Should I tell her that I'd stopped taking my medication?

I didn't want to lie to her. I took another sip of my wine and admitted, "I stopped taking my medication over six months ago."

"What?" Donnita dropped the spoon into the pan and walked toward me. "Dr. Mullin said the seizures will return if you don't take your medication."

"I'm fine," I said stubbornly. "I slowly weaned myself off the medication."

Her eyes narrowed and her voice got louder. "Why didn't you discuss this with me?"

"Because I knew you would react like this," I shot back. "The medication was making me tired. I didn't want to keep going on like that. I decided to see what would happen if I slowly took myself off the medication."

"I'll tell you what's going to happen," she said. "You're going to have seizures again!"

"I have not had a seizure."

"How do you know?" she demanded.

I took a sip of wine. I really didn't want to discuss this any further, but she wasn't finished.

"You need to call Dr. Mullin and tell him what you are doing." She began to pace the floor. "You need to tell Dr. Mullin!"

"No. I'm not calling him!" I raised my voice now too.

"Yes!" she insisted. "He needs to know about this. He told us that you would need to take your medication forever. What happens if you have another seizure when you're driving? You drove to Wenatchee and back home; what if you'd had a seizure driving over Stevens Pass? You could have killed all of us."

I just sat there as she continued.

"Don't you remember what the police and doctors told you after you crashed your car?"

Again, I did not respond.

"I'll tell you what they said: *You are lucky to be alive!*"

"I'm *fine*," I said. "Don't worry."

Donnita's eyes teared up and her face became flushed. I could see the frustration in her eyes. She glared at me and said, "Fine!" Then she stormed out of the kitchen, climbed the stairs, and slammed the bedroom door behind her.

After that night, we never discussed me not taking my medication again.

CHAPTER 101

WHEN I STARTED recruiting at Triad Group, I focused on finding companies willing to pay a fee, and I didn't care about the role. Over those years, I worked on engineering, QA, business development, sales, and marketing roles. I preferred to work on marketing roles versus engineering or QA roles because marketers were natural networkers and would refer me to people who were open to looking at something new—but I always felt it didn't make sense to be picky.

That all changed in 2010, when I started placing people on the marketing team at Marketo. In October of that year, I received an email from Greg Ott, the CMO at Demandbase. He said he'd heard I had placed marketers at Marketo and wanted to speak to me about helping him build his team.

Greg moved to the Bay Area from Seattle, so we had much to talk about. After our first call, I felt I had known him for years. We just clicked. He told me all about Demandbase, then asked me if I would be interested in working on four director-level roles for his team. Of course, I said yes! I ended up placing all four roles for him—and after that, it seemed

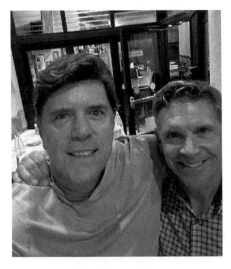

Me and Greg

my name was being circulated around Silicon Valley as "the guy who places top marketers." Over the next few months, I got numerous emails from CMOs looking to build out their marketing teams and CEOs looking to hire VPs of Marketing and CMOs. I decided now was the time to focus on only placing marketers.

At the same time I was placing marketers, I was also getting emails from recently laid-off marketers. A growing theme I kept hearing was that after a new CMO joined their company, they immediately brought over people from their old company.

I had an idea.

I did a search on LinkedIn for everyone on the marketing team at a company where a CMO had recently joined the team. I sent an email to everyone on the marketing team, introducing myself and letting them know that I'd heard a new marketing executive had recently joined their company and would most likely be looking to bring over their own people. It was an effective tactic: over the years, I have pulled a number of people out of companies and placed them in roles before their new VP of Marketing or CMO could replace them with someone from their previous company.

There was always something new to learn.

SINCE I'D MADE a strategic decision to focus only on placing marketers, I decided to update my LinkedIn profile. It now read, *I specialize in placing Director and VP-level Marketing roles (VP/CMO, Product Marketing, Demand Generation, and Corporate Communications) at fast-growing B2B tech companies in Silicon Valley.*

Even though CMOs and CEOs were contacting me to help build their marketing teams, I knew I still had to do some business development. Whenever I noticed companies posting marketing jobs on LinkedIn, Monster, or Craigslist, I would check out the company and see if it was in a similar space to other companies I had recruited for. If it was, I would find out who the hiring manager was and then send them an email, mentioning the big names in their space that I had placed people for. The return on those emails was huge.

I ended up placing eighteen people in 2010, and things did not slow down for me in 2011. At the end of 2011, I once again broke the Triad Group company record for the highest permanent placement billings in a year. I went on to place eighteen people in 2012 and sixteen people in 2013.

I learned a valuable lesson on how to grow your career while placing people at fast-growing startups that would go on to have successful IPOs: Chase companies, not money or titles! If you go to a good company, you will never have to *look* for a job again.

Since I had a great 2011, I finally broke down and traded in my 1998 Toyota Camry, which now had over a hundred thousand miles on it, for a black Infiniti G37. (Of course, I did not buy a new car; I bought a 2009 model with hardly any miles on it.)

I'd always wanted another convertible, but I wasn't sure it was practical given Seattle's weather. After hearing me go back and forth about it for ages, Donnita finally stepped in and said, "You've wanted a convertible for years. Get the convertible."

I listened to her and bought it—and I've never regretted it. I still have that G37 today, and it looks just as pristine as it did the day I bought it.

It was crazy to think that just two years earlier, I'd been so stressed out thinking that we might have made a colossal mistake by overextending and buying a house during the financial crisis. I was glad that even when I was worried about our circumstances, I'd always believed in myself and believed that things would work out. *Just keep moving forward* was my motto, and it had served me well.

CHAPTER 102

WHAT IS YOUR WHY? I constantly hear that question on podcasts and read it in articles almost daily. When I think about my answer, I can say that it has changed from when I first started as a recruiter in 1998. In 1998, the recruiting industry was new to me, and all I cared about was making money (understandable, since I had no money and was deeply in debt). After hitting my stride in 2003, however, I became aware that being a recruiter put me in a position to change people's lives more than just financially.

Over the years, I have helped people get out of toxic companies and placed them in roles where they truly enjoyed going to work every day. I have placed people at companies where I have shortened their commute from an hour's drive to a fifteen-minute bike ride. I have placed people at companies where they have eventually met their true love. I have been able to help my childhood friends' kids land jobs at tech companies right out of college. I have also been able to place people at companies where they've made more money than they could have ever imagined.

One thing I really love is placing people at early-stage startups, because of the opportunity that presents to attain financial freedom.

I caught up with someone in April 2021 whom I'd placed at Coupa a few years after Rob became CEO. I negotiated this person a great salary, plus, I was also able to get him a large number of options—tens of thousands of them. He had worked at Coupa for over four years and had vested his options. I knew Coupa stock had taken off in February, trading at $369 a share, so after we chatted briefly, I cut to the chase: "So, did you sell your Coupa stock?"

"Yep," he said. "I sold almost all my stock when it first hit three hundred dollars a share."

"Congrats!" I said. "I'm so happy for you."

"Thanks," he said. "I need to thank you again for thinking of me for the role."

"You're welcome." I decided to mess with him a little, have some fun. "I have an idea how you can thank me," I proposed. "I'm going to let you pick the color: red or black."

"What? What are you talking about?" he asked.

"Red or black?" I repeated. "Your choice."

"I don't get it," he said.

I let him off the hook. "I'm going to let you pick the color of my new Corvette Stingray," I said, chuckling.

He laughed. "Very funny!"

I never did get my Stingray—but I have received some fantastic gifts from candidates I have placed and CEOs who have hired people from me over the years, including a bottle of extremely rare eighteen-year-old Scotch, a box of steaks from Omaha Steaks, bottles of wine, and more.

The thank-you gifts were great, but it's the thank-you cards that have moved me at a deep level. Like this one: *MK- Thank you for all your support over the years. You've been unwavering in your belief in me—noting that I'd be a CMO, even back when I was a marketing specialist. You believed in me perhaps before I even did. You helped make it happen. Thank you!*

People have told me stories of recruiters who've pressured them to accept an offer. Some recruiters have gone as far as telling a candidate that their firm will not work with them again if they don't take the offer they have in front of them. I could never do that. When I started as a recruiter, I never wanted to be that "pushy sales guy"—and I still feel that way.

About ten years ago, I started letting people know that if they were getting close to an offer from a company, they could let me know the name of the company, and I would let them know if I knew about any "skeletons in the closet." If I knew the previous CMO or the person whose position they were replacing, I would also offer to set up a call with them. I have had people pull themselves out of the interview process and turn down offers after I told them what I knew about a company or after they spoke to an ex-employee. There was no monetary gain for me to do this. I just wanted to make sure someone did not make a colossal mistake and join a lousy company if I could stop it.

After all these years, I think I have figured out my *why*—and I truly believe that I have the greatest job in the world.

CHAPTER 103

Is it better to be lucky than good? Does everything happen for a reason, and we end up where we are supposed to be? Over the years, I have contemplated these two questions. Of course, everyone would love to be good *and* lucky—but if you could only pick one, which would you pick?

Since I'm a sports guy, I look at athletes who have become superstars and won Super Bowl and World Series rings, and I think about what their legacies might have looked like if different organizations had drafted them. Then I look at the superstar athletes who have been the top players in their sports and never won a professional championship.

We all know the amazing NFL quarterback Patrick Mahomes. What would Patrick Mahomes's career look like if the 2017 NFL draft announcement sounded like this: *With the 2nd pick in the 2017 NFL draft, the Chicago Bears select Patrick Mahomes II—quarterback, Texas Tech.* I believe it is safe to say that he would not be wearing three Super Bowl rings. Then you have MLB superstar Mike Trout. Mike Trout is ranked in the top one hundred of the greatest players in MLB history; some of his peers rank him as the greatest player ever. Yet he has played in just three postseason games, all of which his team lost in a three-game Division Series.

So, is Patrick Mahomes just lucky and Mike Trout just unlucky, or did they end up exactly where they were supposed to?

As in professional sports, success at a tech startup depends on being part of a great organization led by a great owner (CEO) and great coaches (executives). You need to be good at what you do, and then you need to sprinkle in some luck. If you are really fortunate, you are in a position to do it multiple times. As a recruiter, I have spoken to people with MBAs from some of the top schools in the country who have had the bad luck of joining small startups that never matured or mid-sized companies that never found their stride. I have also spoken to people who were good but not great who joined small startups that exploded and had huge IPOs, with their stock soaring to over $400 a share.

When the pandemic hit in early 2020, there were companies on the opposite end of the "luck" spectrum. Two companies that come to mind are ZoomandTripActions (rebranded to Navan). In February 2020, Zoom stock was trading at $105 a share. With over one-third of the US employees working from home in May, Zoom stock skyrocketed to $559 a share by October. Zoom had the *perfect* product at the *perfect* time. Unfortunately, TripActions was in a different situation with their products.

As 2019 ended, TripActions had three thousand customers and one thousand employees and raised over $480 million at a valuation of $4 billion. Everything lined up for a massive IPO in 2020. Employees who had been there for over four years were waiting for their big payday. Unfortunately, TripActions had the *wrong* product at the *wrong* time—a business travel platform. In March 2020, TripActions laid off three hundred people, and the global crisis resulted in its revenue dropping to $0.

In a *Forbes* magazine interview, the wildly successful Mark Cuban admitted that his lucky break was exactly that. "Luck is a huge part of everyone's success," he said.

I have to say, I agree. Over the years, I've made some huge placements that fell right into my lap. It was pure luck; all I could do was look to the skies and say, "Thank you, whoever made that happen!"

How the hell do those things happen in our lives? Is it luck? Was it because I was good? Or was it because everything happens for a reason, and I'm exactly where I'm supposed to be?

WHETHER BECAUSE OF luck or something else, business did not slow down for me between 2014 and 2016—but 2017 did not start as well as I had hoped. I had a big fat zero on the whiteboard for Q1. It was one of those quarters where nothing went my way: my candidates all turned down their offers, came in second place, or pulled themselves out of the interview process.

As April approached, I looked forward to going to San Francisco at the end of the month for Marketo's annual conference, Marketing Nation Summit. I would enjoy spending some time with marketers I had placed and executives who had hired marketers from me over the years. And I was especially looking forward to seeing my parents and my buddies Bob and Chris.

Bob and I had met when I started my second year at Cañada Junior College in Redwood City, and we'd hit it off immediately. He lived with his parents and three siblings in Redwood City at the time, and he was Italian, so that meant there was a family dinner on Sunday nights. He invited me to many dinners over the ensuing years, and we became fast friends.

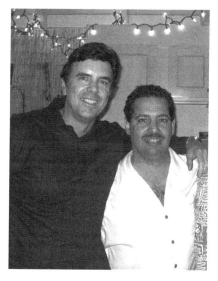

After my surgery in 1998, Donnita and I were in the Bay Area and met Bob and his wife, Karen, for dinner in San Francisco. When Bob saw Donnita, he hugged her tightly and said, "Thank you for taking care of my friend." He and I always made time to have dinner and drinks together when I came to the Bay.

Chris and I had known each other since kindergarten. We'd played

Me and Bob

on the same sports teams (baseball, basketball, and soccer) growing up and played baseball in high school and in junior college. He was the friend I'd called up when I saw Dave Yarnold's name in my inbox and realized I knew him from junior high.

I loved Chris, but since 2013, he'd had a habit of finding the perfect time to bring up a touchy subject I was not interested in discussing with him.

I was ready for him this time, though—or at least I thought I was.

CHAPTER 104

"WHEN ARE YOU GOING to go out on your own?" Chris asked as we walked down a crowded street in San Francisco's financial district.

"Let's go check this place out," I said, hoping to change the subject quickly.

I'd known Chris was going to bring up this subject—he'd done it for the last four years running, after all—but I hadn't thought it would happen so soon during this visit.

I opened the door and entered the space-age interior of Eatsa. Eatsa had opened in 2015 as an automated self-service restaurant where you ordered and paid from iPad kiosks or a mobile app. Your meal was prepared behind wall-mounted glass compartments. Once your meal was ready, a glass compartment lit up with your name.

I ordered the portobello mushroom burrito bowl, and Chris did the same. Within minutes, two glass compartments lit up with our names. We grabbed our food and drinks and went outside to find a table.

Before I could even take a bite of my burrito, Chris started in again.

"How much money do you think you leave on the table every year?"

I took a huge bite of my burrito so I wouldn't have to answer right away. After finally chewing and swallowing my food, I said, "I don't know. I never thought about it. I'm happy where I am."

"How many more years do you think you want to be a recruiter?" he asked.

"I don't know." I shrugged. "Maybe ten more years."

"I bet you leave at least a hundred thousand dollars on the table every year," he said. "That's a million dollars in ten years."

I took another bite of my burrito and swallowed it with difficulty.

"Does your boss give you leads or introductions to executives that might be hiring?" he asked.

I finally gave in and decided to play his little game. "No. Since I joined the company, I have built my whole business by myself. I've built all the relationships with the candidates and opened up all the clients."

"Exactly," he said. "So why are you giving him almost half of what you make?"

"I like where I work," I said. "I have the freedom to make trips like this. I'm not ready to stay home and run my own business. I like going into the office. I like the office atmosphere; it keeps me focused."

Chris finally gave in. "All right. I won't mention it again."

"Really?" I found that hard to believe.

"For now, anyway," he said.

We both laughed, and then we started talking about other things.

WHEN I RETURNED HOME from my trip, I couldn't get one of Chris's comments out of my head: *I bet you leave at least a hundred thousand dollars on the table every year. That's a million dollars in ten years.*

Since I'd billed a big fat $0 in Q1, I had other things to worry about, like having a big Q2.

Happily, things did bounce back for me in Q2; things were looking good in early May. But I still kept returning to what Chris had said. I decided it was time to look at exactly how much I was leaving on the table every year.

CHAPTER 105

I'D BEEN KEEPING a spreadsheet of my quarterly and yearly billings and commissions since my first placement at Triad Group in 2003, so it was easy to calculate how much money I was leaving on the table every year. One night in early May, I sat down and made a spreadsheet to calculate the actual numbers.

I wasn't surprised to see that the actual numbers were exactly what Chris had suggested: a minimum of $100,00 a year.

I still enjoyed working at Triad Group; I didn't really want to leave. Before making any big moves, I decided to speak with Jim to see if I could increase my commission or if he had any other ideas about increasing my pay besides just making more placements.

ON A LATE Friday afternoon in mid-May, after everyone had left the office for the day, I made my way to Jim's office. As I walked down the long hallway, I rehearsed how I wanted to ask for a more significant commission percentage, the same way I had rehearsed asking Jim for the $20,000 for the down payment for our house. Jim's commission structure was very generous compared to other recruiting firms, but I could not get the idea that I was leaving $100,00 a year on the table out of my head.

With my spreadsheet in hand, I knocked on his open door.

Jim looked up from his computer screen. "Yes?"

"You got a minute?"

"Sure." He gestured toward one of the chairs in front of his desk.

When I sat down, he leaned back in his chair and clasped his hands behind his head. "What's going on?"

I shifted in my chair. "First, I want to tell you that I love working here, and I am indebted to you for sticking with me and allowing me to become successful. I am grateful for everything you have done for my family."

Jim did not say a word. He just nodded his head and kept looking at me.

I placed the spreadsheet on his desk. "The other night, I put together a spreadsheet with my billings and commissions from 2010 to 2016 and listed the difference between the two."

I pushed the paper across the desk to Jim. He slowly picked it up and put on his reading glasses.

"I had an idea what those numbers would be every year, but I was surprised when I added up the total number for 2010 to 2016."

Jim sat up and moved his chair closer to his monitor. He looked at the screen on his monitor and then started typing away. He looked at his screen and then down at my piece of paper and scribbled some notes.

After a few minutes, he turned away from his monitor. "Okay. Your numbers for your yearly commissions are off a bit, but the total is close."

I swallowed nervously. "Well, I wanted to talk to you and see if there is anything that can be done to get a bigger piece of my billings. Maybe a higher commission structure?"

"You know I am already paying you a higher commission structure than any other recruiting firm," he said.

"I know," I said. "But if those numbers stay at that rate for the next ten years, that's over a million dollars that I'll leave on the table. I have some close friends who keep telling me I should go out on my own."

"Really?" He frowned. "What do your friends know about running a recruiting business?"

The conversation was not going how I'd hoped. I'd hoped Jim might be open to giving me a more significant piece of the pie, or possibly even making me a partner. Something. Anything.

"I need to get going to meet Ann in Seattle," Jim said. "Let me run some numbers, and let's talk next week." He turned off his computer and grabbed his jacket.

We walked out of his office together. "Have a great weekend," he said before striding away.

"Have a great weekend." I walked back to my office, wondering if I could have handled that conversation better.

CHAPTER 106

BEFORE GOING TO BED on Sunday night, I checked my email and found a message from Jim in my inbox. In it, he reiterated that he was paying me a higher commission than any other recruiting firm, then said it might be time for me to go out on my own. He wanted to meet me on Monday at 3:00 p.m. to discuss some numbers, but he was leaning toward me leaving the company if I was unhappy with my earnings.

I had not been expecting this at all. I showed the email to Donnita, and she was surprised too. I was not ready to leave Triad Group; I didn't want to go.

"Well . . . maybe it *is* time for you to go out on your own," she said.

Maybe Donnita and Chris were right. Maybe it was time for me to do my own thing. Now, I just had to convince myself.

ON MONDAY AT 3:00 P.M., I met with Jim in his office. He went over all the costs associated with my being an employee of Triad Group, making it clear that there was more to it than just billings and commissions, and concluded by saying he could not raise my commission any higher.

I knew I was not ready to leave Triad Group, so I told him I understood and I wanted to stay. Dejected, I left his office and got back to work.

OVER THE NEXT three months, I bounced around the idea of going out on my own. Some days my reaction was a *yes!* and some days it was a big *no!*

One day, while I was driving home from work, one of my favorite songs, "Should I Stay or Should I Go" by the Clash, came on my car radio. I couldn't help but laugh; the timing couldn't have been more perfect, given what I was going through.

On one of the days that I was feeling positive about going out on my own, I did a little exercise: I wrote down all the costs that would be associated with going out on my own. It seemed like they would actually be minimal: a LinkedIn subscription, a Bullhorn (ATS) subscription, a G

Suite subscription, building a website, a business license and other legal documents, and a QuickBooks subscription. I would also have to get medical insurance for me, Donnita, and Natalie, of course, but when I did the numbers, I realized that paying for insurance out of pocket wouldn't cost me much more than I paid at Triad Group.

This idea was starting to feel like it had legs.

ON A RAINY Saturday afternoon a week later, I sat down with a yellow legal pad and wrote what I titled "A Day at Triad Group." It started with me getting up at seven, getting ready for work, and getting out the door by eight to ensure I made it to the office before nine. Once in the office, I said good morning to Kelli, who wore many "Triad hats," including the role of receptionist. After I walked down the hall and said good morning to my fellow recruiters, I entered my office. After I raised my stand-up desk and turned on my computer, it was time to get some coffee. Once in the kitchen, I placed my lunch—which Donnita made for me every single day—in the refrigerator. After pouring myself a big cup of coffee, I returned to my office.

Once I was back at my office, it was time to get to work—finding candidates for open roles, setting up interviews, opening up new clients, and closing deals. When 1:00 p.m. rolled around, I went downstairs to the gym to work out or walked the stairs for a while. After returning from my workout, I ate my lunch, worked until 6:30 p.m., and then made the hour-long commute home. This had been my routine in the office since joining Triad Group in November 2001.

After doing this little exercise, I realized that I was essentially paying for a very expensive WeWork office with all the money I was leaving on the table.

IN LATE AUGUST, I had another meeting with Jim and let him know that I had decided it was time for me to move on. He was not upset that I was leaving; I think he'd known for a while that I would eventually go out on my own.

Of course, Chris was the first person I called to say, "I just resigned!"

My last day at Triad Group was Friday, September 15, 2017. Since I loved working with everyone in the office, it was tough to say goodbye, but I knew I had to do this. When Jim had sent out a company email earlier in the week to inform everyone I was leaving and my last day would be the fifteenth, one of my fellow recruiters had walked into my office, hugged me, and said, "It's about fucking time! Congrats, dude!"

Jim put together a company lunch at Maggiano's in downtown Bellevue on my last day to celebrate my sixteen years at Triad Group. It was fun to hear my coworkers share stories about working with me, and they even roasted me a bit on some of the funny things that had happened during my time at Triad Group. It was a great sendoff.

After lunch, I boxed up my belongings, hugged all my fellow employees goodbye, and drove home. From here on out, I would be on my own.

CHAPTER 107

ON SEPTEMBER 18, the radar sound effect from my iPhone alarm bounced off the bathroom walls. It was time to get up for my first day at King Recruiting, Inc. After turning off my alarm, I changed into my workout gear and headed down the hall to the media room for a workout. After a workout and showering, I changed into my work clothes: a white T-shirt and gray sweatpants.

In 1999, my cousin John had moved from the Bay Area to Santa Monica, California, to begin his new job as an account executive at KTLA television station. Since I was living in LA at the time, he'd asked me if I could help him and his girlfriend move into their apartment.

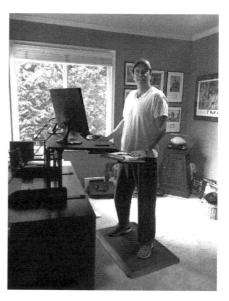

As we carried boxes into the new place, John's girlfriend turned to me and said, "John told me that you are a recruiter. My father is a recruiter."

"That's cool," I said. "Does your father work for a big recruiting firm?"

"He did for over twenty years," she said, "until he finally decided to go out on his own seven years ago. Now he works out of his house."

King Recruiting – First day

"Does he like working from home?"

"Yeah, he does. He said the best part is he could wear his pajamas to work if he really wanted to." She laughed. "He usually wears sweatpants and a T-shirt, which is pretty close."

"Wow!" I shook my head in admiration. "I wish I could do that someday."

I never thought that eighteen years later, I too would be a successful recruiter running his own business from home in sweatpants and a T-shirt.

Look at me now, I thought as I "commuted" down the stairs to my office.

ABOUT A WEEK before I "officially" started King Recruiting, Inc., I'd emailed people I had worked with over the years, notifying them that I was leaving Triad Group and giving them my new contact info and a link to my website. I'd received a ton of supportive, encouraging replies.

A week before going out on my own, I'd also exported my LinkedIn connections into a spreadsheet and imported them into Bullhorn (ATS), bought a QuickBooks subscription, and created a Gmail account for King Recruiting. I was ready to rock and roll!

I had built strong relationships and a strong personal brand over the last fifteen years, so I wasn't worried about opening new clients. Also, Triad Group did not have a noncompete, so I could continue to work with the clients I'd had there.

Getting my first new client, a crypto company, took only a week. One of the VPs at the company had heard about me and wanted to retain me for the VP of Marketing search. I sent my first King Recruiting invoice on October 3, 2017. A few weeks later, I was retained by two other companies for VP of Marketing roles.

My first placement happened two months later, on December 6, when I placed a Director of Product Marketing at a Bellevue, Washington, startup called Adaptiva—which was especially cool because I'd known the CEO, Jim Souders, for years; our daughters had played on the same select softball team together in 2011.

I ended the year with my placement at Adaptiva and four retainers. I was excited when the checks arrived and I got to deposit them into my checking account without leaving any money on the table.

I was looking forward to 2018.

CHAPTER 108

In April 2018, I joined David Lewis on his DemandGen Radio podcast, *Methods and Technologies for Driving Growth*, as his fiftieth guest. The episode title was "How Much Money is Marketing Earning These Days?"

This was the first time I had been invited to be a guest on a podcast, and I had a blast—and when I listened to the episode later, I was happy with how David had edited our conversation. I posted the link on LinkedIn, and I was pleasantly surprised by the comments from listeners.

Two days after the episode was released, I was relaxing on the sofa watching a movie with Donnita when my cell phone rang. When I saw that it was David, I told Donnita that I needed to take the call. We paused the movie and I walked into the kitchen.

"Hello?" I said.

"Hello, Michael. It's David. Sorry to call you on the weekend."

"No worries. What's up?"

"You're probably wondering why I'm calling."

"Are you calling to see how my weekend is going?" I chuckled.

"Funny. No. I'm calling to let you know that your podcast is going through the roof! It may end up being one of my top podcasts."

"Really!" I was pleased, but I didn't think I could take the credit. "I have to tell you, I'm not surprised. I don't think it has as much to do with me as it does with the title you gave the episode."

"I'm sure the title helped," he said, "but you had something to do with it. Are you going to be in town for the Marketo Summit?"

"I am," I said. "And I registered for the DemandGen party on Monday night at the Battery Club."

"Perfect! I'll see you at the party. Have a great night."

"Thanks, you too."

I walked back to the family room with a spring in my step.

BE THERE WHEN I RETURN

— — —

IN EARLY 2018, I decided it was time to get some King Recruiting swag, so I ordered a batch of baseball hats (white and black) with my company name and logo on them, along with a few golf shirts, T-shirts, and a jacket and backpack.

Monday night, April 30, I arrived at the Battery Club in San Francisco dressed in black jeans, a black T-shirt, and a black Eddie Bauer softshell jacket with KING RECRUITING and my logo embroidered on the left chest. I was also rocking a black-and-orange backpack that proudly displayed my company name and logo.

The Battery Club is located at 717 Battery Street—hence the name. It is an invite-only social club with a restaurant, fourteen guest rooms, and an indoor/outdoor penthouse with amazing views of the Bay Bridge and the Transamerica Pyramid building. The party was at the penthouse.

As I exited the elevator and walked through the crowded room, I noticed David Lewis off to the side with a small group of people. He spotted me and waved me over.

As I approached, the people he was speaking with looked at my face and then down at the logo on my jacket. Before I reached him, two guys approached me and said, "Michael, how are you doing? Loved the podcast."

"Thanks!"

I shook hands with the two guys, and they introduced themselves. After a moment, I excused myself and made my way to David, whom I gave a big hug.

"How are you doing?" I asked.

"Good," he said. "I feel your podcast might just be number one by the end of the week."

"Really?"

"Yes, and it's not because of the podcast's title," he said, giving me a nudge.

I enjoyed a drink with David and then walked around the room to say hi to everyone I knew there—people I had placed, people who had hired candidates from me, and people I had met over the years as a recruiter.

I'd started the day with my backpack stuffed with white and black King Recruiting hats; by night's end, my backpack was empty.

BY THE END of the week, my podcast had not quite gotten to number one; it settled in at number two behind an episode with Steve Lucas, Marketo's CEO. But this would not be the last time I was invited to be a guest on a podcast. David Lewis asked me back again a year later, and over the next few years I was also invited to participate in virtual happy hours and even a fireside chat to conclude ActiveCampaign's virtual event *This Just Works*.

With the podcasts and my activity on LinkedIn, I started to get more and more referrals for VP of Marketing and CMO searches, plus referrals to CMOs who wanted me to find them VPs and Directors of Demand Generation, Product Marketing, and Corporate Marketing. I was busier than I could have ever imagined I would be.

I'd meant what I'd said to Chris over burritos: I'd never thought about going out alone in the past because I wasn't sure I wanted to work alone at home. But after working from home for a year, I was surprised to find that I didn't miss the energy of working in an office. I loved that I could take a break and go for a walk or go up to the media room and get in a quick workout anytime I felt like it.

If you asked me what the best part of working from home is, though?

I have a secretary with benefits. (Donnita is going to kill me for writing that!)

I had a great first full year on my own, and things did not slow down for me in 2019.

I was building momentum and looking forward to a huge 2020.

CHAPTER 109

ON MONDAY, MARCH 19, 2020, California governor Gavin Newson issued a stay-at-home order to protect the health and well-being of all Californians. By March 31, there were 192,301 documented coronavirus cases, and the virus had killed 5,334 people in the United States, according to Johns Hopkins University's Coronavirus Resource Center.

By the end of March, the tech industry had cut more than 40,000 jobs. In a single week in early May, Uber announced it would slash 3,700 positions, Airbnb said it would cut 1,900, and Lyft fired or furloughed more than 1,000 people.

Fortunately, not all tech companies were having layoffs. Companies whose products benefited people who were stuck at home—Facebook, Zoom, Peloton, Salesforce, DocuSign, Microsoft, Netflix, Amazon, DoorDash, Apple, Shopify, Google, and HelloFresh, to name a handful— exploded and went on hiring sprees.

For my business, hiring at B2B tech startups based in the San Francisco Bay Area slowed down from May to September. I did not make a placement in Q3. I was financially okay, however, as I had listened to my mom's sound advice—*"Make sure you save money for a rainy day."* Well, the rainy days (and months) were here.

In August, things started to loosen up, and HR departments, CEOs, and CMOs were open to having me work on searches again. But they told me I could only work on the roles if I lowered my fees. Since this was the third tech downturn I was experiencing, I knew how this worked. I did what I had to do and lowered my fee.

What I wasn't expecting was something I began to hear from CMOs and CEOs during this time: "We aren't planning on returning to an office anytime soon, so we are leaning toward hiring someone outside of the Bay Area. I'm sure they will be a lot cheaper."

Oh shit! I thought.

Since starting in the recruiting business in 1998, I had only worked with tech companies headquartered in the San Francisco Bay Area. Before the pandemic, all my clients had mostly insisted on employees being in the office daily. I didn't know anyone in the industry outside of the Bay Area.

It was time to expand my network.

I immediately jumped on LinkedIn and contacted director and VP-level marketers at B2B SaaS companies outside the Bay Area. Since I had built a strong brand, I created new connections fairly quickly, and soon I had built a robust list of marketers outside the Bay Area. Over the next two years, I placed candidates who lived in New York, Pittsburgh, North Carolina, Utah, Oregon, San Diego, and Los Angeles at a number of clients headquartered in the Bay Area.

Things picked up for me in September, and I had a strong Q4. I had some great candidates deep in the interview process. It looked like January 2021 would be starting off great.

CHAPTER 110

January 2021. I had been seizure-free since after my surgery in 1998 and had been off my medication since 2010 without any complications. I'd just finished enjoying one of my favorite dishes for dinner at the "Donnita Café"—linguini and clams.

After taking the last sip of my Washington chardonnay, I rose from my seat and stretched. "I'm going to head upstairs to take a hot Epsom salt bath."

"Enjoy!" Donnita said.

Once upstairs in the bathroom, I plugged in my iPhone, opened Pandora, clicked on Michael Kiwanuka Radio, and filled the tub.

After soaking in the tub for about thirty minutes, I had worked up a good sweat, and it was time to get out. I stood up fast and stepped out of the tub, then bent over and started wiping the soap suds off my legs—and then everything went dark.

Donnita was at the sink, washing dishes, when a loud thump from the ceiling above her caught her attention. She turned off the faucet, listened for a second, and then called out, "Michael!"

No response.

"Michael!" she shouted again.

Still no response, so she went to the bottom of the stairs and yelled, "Michael! Are you okay?"

"Yeah . . . I'm okay," I finally answered.

Donnita was still worried, so she came upstairs to check on me. She found me sitting on the stone floor of the bathroom, steam rising off my upper body and head.

"Are you okay?" she asked.

"I'm fine. I bent over to wipe the soap suds off my leg, got a little dizzy, and fell. I'm okay."

"Let me get you a cold washcloth to cool you off." She grabbed a washcloth from a cabinet, ran cold water over it, and started to walk toward me.

Without warning, I flung my head back and slammed the back of my head on the stone floor—so hard that my head bounced off the floor, scaring Donnita—and started to make a moaning sound. My eyes were wide open, staring at the ceiling, as my forearms extended into a fencing response (a pose where one arm is bent toward the body and the other is outstretched; it occurs when severe brain trauma has been suffered).

"Natalie!" Donnita screamed as she grabbed a towel and covered my private parts.

As she picked up the phone and dialed 911, Natalie came running into the bathroom. "What happened?" she asked.

"Your father hit his head on the floor," Donnita explained. "I'm on with 911."

Natalie sat down next to me. My arms slowly came down from the fencing position and were now lying at my sides. My eyes were still wide open and fixed on the ceiling. I didn't blink.

"Michael!" Donnita called out.

I did not respond. My face and body started to turn pale.

"Wake up, Dad! Please wake up, Dad!" Natalie pleaded. She started to cry as she lightly tapped my face.

"He's not responding—I think he's dead!" Donnita frantically yelled into the phone.

Just then, I started to come out of it. I slowly blinked my eyes; I looked around the bathroom. As I tried to get my bearings, I heard Donnita's voice. I sat up gingerly and saw Donnita in front of me, the phone pressed to her ear.

"Mom!" Natalie called out. "Dad is sitting up!"

I was surprised she was there sitting next to me, and was confused to see tears rolling down her red cheeks.

"He is coming out of it! He's coming out of it! He is sitting up now," Donnita said with excitement. "Yes, please send an ambulance."

That got my attention. "Ambulance? No, I don't need an ambulance. I'm fine."

"Dad, you hit your head, and you're bleeding," Natalie said as she wiped tears from her face and showed me a small blood stain on the washcloth Donnita had placed under my head.

"I'm fine—I'm okay!" I said to Donnita.

She covered the phone with her hand. "You are *not* okay!" She returned to her conversation with the 911 operator, trying to regain her composure. "Thank you," she said into the phone. After she hung up, she turned back to me. "The ambulance is on its way. You need to put on some clothes."

I slowly got to my feet and put on a pair of sweatpants and a T-shirt. I sat on the bed with Donnita, drank some water, and tried to think about what had just happened to me.

The sound of the doorbell echoed through the house, startling me.

"The ambulance is here!" Natalie called out from downstairs.

"Stay here," Donnita told me before going downstairs to greet them.

Moments later, she walked back into the bedroom, two EMTs right behind her. "How are you doing?" one of the EMTs asked me.

"I'm fine!" I said.

"You are *not* fine!" Donnita said with an edge to her voice. "You slammed your head on the stone."

"Are you okay with going downstairs?" the other EMT asked.

"Yep," I said. I stood up and followed them down the stairs to the living room, where we sat on the sofa so they could examine me.

The first EMT checked the back of my head. The cut was small and was not bleeding. He cleaned my wound and asked me questions to see if I had a concussion: "What is your name?"; "Where are you?"; "What day is it?"; "What year is it?"; "Can you count from ten backward?"

As I answered his questions, the second EMT spoke with Donnita, getting my history and the story of what had just happened. Curious, I kept one ear open, listening to what Donnita had to say.

First, she went through the details of what had just happened; then she paused, and her voice cracked as she said, "He was diagnosed with epilepsy in 1992 and had surgery in 1997. He has been seizure-free since the surgery. Do you think he had a seizure?"

"I don't know," the EMT said. "Does he take medication for his epilepsy?"

I looked at Donnita; she glared back at me.

"He stopped taking his medication in 2010," she said, shaking her head.

"I would suggest taking him in and getting him checked out," the EMT said.

Did I have a seizure? I wondered, my heart in my throat. *If I did, is it because I stopped taking my medication? Am I going to go back to having multiple seizures a day?*

I snapped out of it when the EMT asked, "Any nausea?"

I quickly responded, "Nope." But I was not being 100 percent honest with him. As I'd walked down the stairs a few moments earlier, my throat and mouth had started to get dry—but it had only lasted for a minute, so I didn't think I needed to tell him.

The EMT who was speaking with Donnita made his way over to me. "Since you hit your head on the ground and you were unconscious, you probably should go in and get a CT scan just to make sure everything is okay," he said.

My stubborn personality kicked in then. "I feel fine," I said. "I don't think I need a CT scan."

"You really should go in and get checked out," Donnita pleaded with me.

"I'm fine," I said, my jaw set.

"Look at your wife's and daughter's faces," the EMT said. "They are very concerned for you."

I looked over at Donnita. Her face still showed signs of trauma; just thirty minutes earlier, she thought she'd watched me die on the bathroom floor. I turned my head to look up at Natalie, standing on the stairs. She wiped tears from her face.

My heart ached for them both, but I still didn't want to go to the hospital. "I'm fine," I said again. "I don't want to go to the hospital."

Donnita knew how stubborn I could be; she didn't push the issue further.

"Okay," the EMT said, frowning. "I'm going to need you to sign some paperwork."

I signed the paperwork they presented me with—which stated that I'd been informed I should go to the hospital for additional testing, but I'd declined—and the EMTs wished me luck and left.

BE THERE WHEN I RETURN

- - -

AFTER THE EMTs left the house, I waited about a minute, then got off the sofa and headed toward the family room. As I entered the family room, my throat and mouth suddenly became parched. "Oh shit!" I said, and sprinted for the bathroom.

I didn't make it to the toilet on time; I threw up on the floor.

Donnita entered the bathroom. "I told you! You have a concussion!"

I leaned up against the bathroom wall. "I'm sorry—I'll clean it up," I said, taking a deep breath.

"No!" she snapped. "I'll clean it up. Just go wash your face and sit down."

After I washed my face, I grabbed a Gatorade from the refrigerator and sat on the sofa, still in denial that anything might be wrong with me.

After Donnita cleaned the bathroom, the three of us watched a movie together. During the movie, I could feel Donnita's and Natalie's eyes on me, watching and waiting to see if anything else would happen.

Nothing did, and when the movie ended, we all headed upstairs to go to bed.

I FELL ASLEEP quickly that night. But at some point in the middle of the night, I suddenly woke up. I frantically looked around the room. My breathing accelerated.

My movement in the bed woke up Donnita. "What's wrong?" she asked.

For what felt like a long time, I couldn't catch my breath. When I finally did, I said, "I had the strangest dream. It was morning, and you leaned over to give me a good morning kiss, and I was dead."

"What?" she asked, a note of fear in her voice.

"I think I should go to Kaiser in the morning and get a CT scan," I said.

"I agree," she said. "It would be best if you got checked out. I don't think you realize how hard you hit your head on the floor."

"I probably should have let the EMTs take me to the hospital to get checked out," I admitted.

"Yes, you should have," she said. "You need to stop being so stubborn."

"I know . . . I know." I sighed.

You would think I would have learned my lesson in 1992, when I didn't listen to Donnita and Tim after they told me something was wrong with me. I should have seen a doctor then, and I should have gone with the EMTs and had a CT scan.

I hugged and kissed Donnita and held her tightly as we fell asleep.

AT 10:00 A.M. THE NEXT DAY, I had a CT scan at Kaiser Permanente Medical Center in Bellevue. Thankfully, the tests came back negative. There was no bleeding or excessive fluid in my brain, and the structure of my skull remained intact.

The doctor could not say if I'd had a seizure or not, and we will never know, but that night will be etched in Donnita's and Natalie's memory forever.

I took this experience as a sign that it was not my time. Since my thirties, I have been fascinated by people who have done things that should have killed them and yet somehow have survived, while others have died. In 1992, for example, Slash, lead guitarist of Guns N' Roses, overdosed in a hotel in San Francisco on a speedball—a deadly mixture of cocaine and heroin. He experienced a cardiac arrest for eight minutes, died, was revived, and is still with us. In 1993, in contrast, actor River Phoenix also did a speedball and died outside the Viper Room on Sunset Boulevard in LA. Why did River die and not Slash? I'm still trying to figure out how Keith Richards is still alive when on the news every day I hear about a tree falling on someone and killing them or a wrong-way driver killing a young couple and their children.

As someone who has been told by the police that I was fortunate to be alive after having a seizure while driving and crashing my car into the trees, and as someone who slammed my head on the bathroom floor, lay unconscious, and turned pale, I genuinely believe we are born with a "time stamp" (day and time) for our death. On that day and time, you will pass. It could be walking across the street, it could be in a car or an airplane, but it will happen.

I'm glad my "time stamp" did not turn out to read April 30, 1996, 5:30 p.m., or January 27, 2021, 8:15 p.m.

CHAPTER 111

BESIDES MY SCARE in January of 2021, the year started off great. I made over $250K in Q1, and things did not slow down for me as the year progressed. VCs were handing out large checks to fast-growing startups, and post-IPO companies were flush with cash.

That meant one thing: *Grow, grow, grow!*

And this growth mentality was not just for startups and post-IPO companies. That year, big tech companies in the Bay Area went on a hiring spree. Between 2020 and 2021, Salesforce went from 49,000 employees to 56,606, Facebook went from 58,604 to 71,970, and Google went from 135,301 to 156,500.

I was so busy in 2021 that I asked Natalie, now in her twenties, the same question at least two times a week: "You sure you don't want to be a recruiter?"

After she finally gave me a stern "No!" I stopped asking—and I didn't blame her. If someone had asked me if I wanted to be a recruiter in my early twenties, I'm sure I would have had the same response.

I thought about hiring someone to help me find candidates, but I decided against it. I didn't want to have to manage someone and worry about whether they were looking for the right candidates for my clients.

Since companies still had the mindset of "grow at all costs," there was a shortage of qualified candidates looking for new roles. Companies were aware of this supply-demand gap in the labor market, so they knew they had to make quick decisions with candidates. Since some small startups had raised rounds of over $50 million, they had the resources to compete with larger startups for talent. They were overpaying for talent.

Everyone knew this craziness could not last forever, but no one knew exactly when things would come crashing down. It seemed the companies didn't care; they just kept hiring and hiring.

When Q4 started, I had already made $800K for the year. I only needed to make $200K in Q4 to hit a number I would never have thought possible even a year earlier: $1 million.

Some people think Q4 is a slow recruiting time because of the holidays in November and December, but over the years it has frequently been one of my biggest quarters. This year was no exception; my Q4 was just as busy as my previous three quarters, and I made a placement on November 17 that put me over $1 million for the year. Now it was time to get ready for Thanksgiving.

SINCE MOVING INTO our house in 2009, we'd hosted Thanksgiving for Donnita's side of the family. The number of people who showed up grew over the years and finally tapped out at thirty-five people. At this year's celebration we had twenty family members, and as usual Donnita did all the cooking. Appetizers: brie en croute, deviled eggs, and crudité platter. Dinner: turkey, ham, dressing, green beans, mashed potatoes and gravy, spinach and hot sausage (my grandma's recipe), sweet potatoes, and cranberry sauce (not from a can).

As the last of our guests slowly made their way out the front door with full bellies and leftovers in their hands, I sat down to enjoy a nice glass of the eighteen-year-old Glenmorangie a CEO had gifted me a few years earlier.

The prior three years had been crazy for our family. My dad had passed away in 2019. I'd broken my right ankle in 2019. Donnita's mom had passed away earlier in 2021. My mom's health was poor and not improving. Donnita had suffered two medical emergencies in the last two years: a dime-sized hole in her large intestine in 2020, and a detached retina in October of this year. We needed some time to get away and relax.

Luckily, we already had something booked: a two-week vacation for our family of three in Cabo San Lucas. We were all looking forward to leaving for Cabo on December 4.

CHAPTER 112

ON DECEMBER 11, I made my way to the bar by the pool at our resort in Cabo San Lucas and ordered a Corona. I took a big sip of my beer, walked to a lounge chair, and lay down.

It was the beginning of week two in Cabo for us. I had already played two rounds of golf—at Quivira and Cabo Real; we had experienced some great restaurants, Flora Farms and Sunset Monalisa; and we had just come back from a fantastic snorkeling trip where we'd seen whales and dolphins. Now I needed to just chill. This was, after all, a vacation.

After finishing my beer, I got up and strolled to the edge of the pool area, where a picturesque cliff afforded me a panoramic view of the stunning sandy beach. I could see Donnita and Natalie down there, playfully dipping their toes into the inviting waters of the Gulf of California, their faces wreathed in smiles.

I gazed at the Arch of Cabo San Lucas, illuminated by the radiant sun above. I took a deep breath and tilted my head back, allowing the sun to caress my face. I closed my eyes and reflected on the journey that had brought me to this moment.

I thought back to that sunny day in Los Angeles in February of 1997 when I stood on the roof of my apartment, feeling so lost and hopeless. I thought back to 1992 in LA, when I had my first seizure in my apartment. I thought about how blessed I was to have found Donnita before my life was turned upside-down. I thought about how blessed I was to have survived my car crash and not killed an innocent bystander. I thought about when we moved to Seattle for a new job and I didn't make a single placement in over a year.

There had been a number of times in my life when I'd thought about giving up, but I never had. I couldn't. Above all, I had always been determined not to give up.

I truly believe that the most underrated quality is determination. It is more important than having a solid network.

I looked down at Donnita and Natalie as they swam in the ocean below, and reflected on all the people who had come into my life and changed it for the better. Would I have transferred to St. Ignatius without meeting Patty Martin? No! Would I have gotten into acting and modeling if I hadn't ended up in Brother Matthew's class at St. Mary's? No! Would I have met Donnita if I had not sent that note to her at the Hard Rock in LA? No! Would I have gotten into recruiting if I had not run into Calvin at the Griffith Park Golf Course? Definitely not! Would I have met Jim Mercer if I had given up on looking for a recruiting job? No way!

We really do meet everyone in our lives for a reason.

I thought about how blessed I was to have had that surgery at UCLA that cured my epilepsy. How fortunate we were to buy our first and second house before the Seattle-area housing market exploded.

I pondered the timeless wisdom of one of my mother's favorite sayings, "Good things happen to good people."

Tears rolled off my face and fell to the sand below.

When I started recruiting, my goal was to make $100K in a year. Now I could make $100K in one placement. Since going out on my own at the end of 2017, I have made more money than I ever imagined was possible. As Chris always reminds me, "You should have listened to me years ago."

It still amazes me how everything has fallen into place for me over the last twenty-plus years. I have told Donnita many times that I sometimes have this weird feeling that this whole journey has been nothing but a dream—that one day I will wake up next to her on a beach in LA and it will be 1997 again, a few days before I'm set to start my testing at UCLA.

If this is a dream, I hope I never wake up.

There is no such thing as a straight path in our lives. Moving through this world can be chaotic, harsh, and unpredictable. But when we open our hearts and eyes to new opportunities and challenges, we will always end up exactly where we should be.

So, I'll leave you with these last words of advice, which I mean from the bottom of my heart:

Keep moving forward. Never give up.

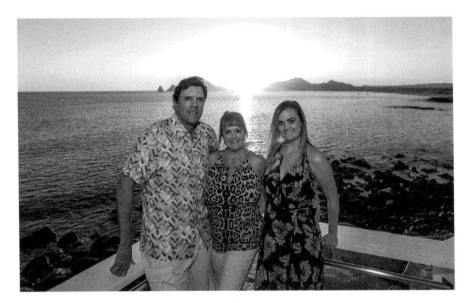

Cabo

ACKNOWLEDGMENTS

THE DECISION TO dive into writing this book has been quite the adventure. It's been a journey filled with introspection and reminiscing, made possible by the shared memories and support of my buddies Tim and Dave, my ever-encouraging parents, and my wonderful wife, Donnita. Together, we've revisited the highs and lows of my early experiences with epilepsy, and I'm incredibly grateful for their contributions throughout this process.

My heartfelt thanks go to Dr. Espy, whose expertise, compassion, and unwavering support guided me through the daunting journey of epilepsy diagnosis and treatment. From the moment you identified my epilepsy, you gave me more than just answers—you gave me a path forward. Thank you for being a crucial part of my story.

I owe immense gratitude to the exceptional staff at UCLA, particularly Dr. Jerome Engel Jr., Dr. Itzhak Fried, Dr. Paul Mullin, Dr. Igor Fineman, Dr. James Forage, and my nurse specialist, Dr. Sandra Dewar, whose unwavering care and expertise not only transformed my life but also shaped the person I am today. Thank you for everything.

To my dear friends—Tom, Matt, Kelvin, and Justin—thank you for your invaluable feedback on my early drafts. A special thank-you to Joshua Mohr for his dedication in helping me shape a compelling story. To Krissa Lagos, my exceptional copyeditor, thank you for your meticulous work in bringing my story to life on the page. To Chas Hoppe, thanks for coming up with the perfect title. And to Natalia Olbinski and Tabitha Lahr for designing a beautiful cover.

Special thanks to Brooke Warner, Addison Gallegos, and the entire editorial team at SparkPress for their invaluable guidance throughout the publishing journey. Without your expertise and support, navigating this process would have been incredibly daunting.

It tugs at my soul that my book was not completed before the passing of Jim Dekker and my parents. Jim, a cherished figure in my life—my high school baseball coach, an English teacher, and a published author—was the first person I reached out to upon finishing my initial draft. He readily agreed to review the first one hundred pages, insisting on traditional methods, requiring me to mail him the printed pages. His feedback proved invaluable, urging me forward with each suggestion. Meanwhile, my parents held steadfast pride in my endeavor, eagerly awaiting updates on my progress. I'd share chapters with my mother, relishing her encouragement. Sadly, the completion of the book came too late for them to share in its publication.

Finally, this book would never have come to fruition without the love and support of my wife, Donnita, and my daughter, Natalie. Your unwavering belief in me has been my guiding light throughout this endeavor. Thank you for standing by my side—I cherish and love you both immensely!

ABOUT THE AUTHOR

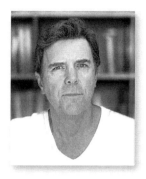

MICHAEL KING WAS born in San Francisco and raised in Daly City, California. He is an epilepsy survivor and the founder and CEO of King Recruiting, Inc. Michael is an avid sports fan. When he's not placing marketers at top tech companies in Silicon Valley, you can find him chasing a little white ball on the golf course. Today, he lives in Sammamish, Washington, with his wife and daughter.

Follow Michael at www.michaeltking.com

Looking for your next great read?

We can help!

Visit www.gosparkpress.com/next-read
or scan the QR code below for a list
of our recommended titles.

SparkPress is an independent boutique publisher
delivering high-quality, entertaining, and engaging
content that enhances readers' lives, with a special
focus on commercial and genre fiction.